Progress in Behavioral Social Work

Progress in Behavioral Social Work

Bruce A. Thyer
Walter W. Hudson
Editors

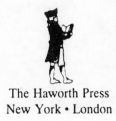

The Haworth Press
New York • London

10-13-89

Progress in Behavioral Social Work has also been published as *Journal of Social Service Research*, Volume 10, Numbers 2/3/4, Winter 1986/Spring/Summer 1987.

The Haworth Press, Inc., 12 West 32 Street, New York, NY 10001
EUROSPAN/Haworth, 3 Henrietta Street, London WC2E 8LU England

Library of Congress Cataloging-in-Publication Data

Progress in behavioral social work.

Has also been published as Journal of social service research, v. 10, no. 2/3/4, Winter 1986/Spring/Summer 1987.
Bibliography: p.
1. Psychiatric social work. 2. Behavior modification. I. Thyer, Bruce A. II. Hudson, Walter W.
HV689.P684   1987   362.2'0425   87-19819
ISBN 0-86656-656-2

Progress in Behavioral Social Work

Journal of Social Service Research
Volume 10, Numbers 2/3/4

CONTENTS

Progress in Behavioral Social Work

Progress in Behavioral Social Work: An Introduction

The field of behavioral social work, barely two decades old, has rapidly become an important and influential perspective among the various schools of social work intervention. Over 50 textbooks (Thyer, 1985) and hundreds of articles (Thyer, 1981) are currently available that describe, test and validate the efficacy of behavioral approaches when applied to problem areas of concern to professional social workers. The diversity of practice techniques, practice modalities (individual, group, family, community, etc.) and substantive problem areas (mental health, health care, child welfare, substance abuse, etc.) associated with behavioral social work has made it somewhat difficult to precisely distinguish behavioral approaches to social work practice from alternative theoretical positions. Accordingly, we offer the following as our generic definition of behavioral social work:

> Behavioral social work is the informed use, by professional social workers, of interventive techniques based upon empirically-derived learning theories that include but are not limited to, operant conditioning, respondent conditioning, and observational learning. Behavioral social workers may or may not subscribe to the philosophy of behaviorism.

We believe that this definition clarifies several issues. First, behavioral social work is an *informed* approach to intervention that is conducted by social workers who use relevant theoretical knowledge to guide their development of an intervention plan.

Accordingly, practitioners who inadvertently or through practice wisdom find simple reinforcement techniques useful in working with clients would not be considered to be practicing behavioral social work.

All behavioral social work is informed and guided by empirically established principles of human learning. Although this may not be explicit, in practice behavioral social workers should always be able to provide a theoretical rationale for the major components of their treatment plans. At present, behavioral and social science has validated many of the principles associated with operant, respondent and observational learning theories. We recognize that this is an evolving process. Fifty years ago there was no such field known as operant conditioning and we can expect that fifty years hence our understanding of the complexities of human behavior will render present formulations obsolete. For example, the distinction between operant and respondent behavior may become subsumed under a single, more comprehensive, mechanism of learning; observational learning may prove to be a special case of operant conditioning; or certain cognitive theories may need to be added to our list. We eagerly await these advances in behavioral science knowledge.

The final sentence in our definition highlights an important distinction which is often overlooked by commentators in the field. The application of knowledge from the science of human behavior (variously known as applied behavior analysis, behavior therapy or behavior modification) is quite distinct from *behaviorism* which is a *philosophy* of the science of behavior (Skinner, 1974). Social workers may make use of behavioral approaches in their practice without subscribing to the philosophical perspectives associated with behaviorism. This would be analogous to the behavioral social worker who makes skilled use of empathy, warmth, and genuineness, but does not adhere to the additional tenets associated with client-centered therapy or the philosophy of secular humanism.

Another salient characteristic of behavioral social work is its general focus upon conceptualizing the origins of client and societal problems from a strongly *environmental* perspective, as opposed to a mentalistic, personality, intraspsychic or dispositional one. This is usually formulated in terms of an individual's learning history, or of ongoing environmental contingencies of rein-forcement and punishment that affect a person, group, family, or community. Such a perspective avoids the problem of circular reasoning commonly associated with purported dispositional ex-planations, avoids attributing blame to an already overburdened client, and generates parsimonious explanations of social work problems that are capable of being empirically tested. This envi-ronmental approach is congruent with the long standing advo-cacy of a person-in-environment perspective for social work practice, perhaps more so than any other theoretical perspective (Thyer, 1987).

As a profession we can take pride in the recent reviews of the effectiveness of social work practice which indicate that social workers are helping clients and larger systems to ameliorate sig-nificant problems of personal and social importance (Reid & Hanrahan, 1982; Rubin, 1985; Videka-Sherman, 1985). It is no coincidence that the majority of the well-controlled group out-come studies of social work which demonstrate such a positive impact are behavioral in their orientation. For example, by our count, 18 of the 29 articles reviewed by Reid and Hanrahan (1982) were based upon behavioral interventions.

It is somewhat ironic that concurrent with this emergence of an empirical basis for social work practice (evidence only available through the use of operationally-defined client problems, struc-tured social work interventions and sophisticated research de-signs) vocal opponents of these traditional methods of science are suggesting that we abandon such approaches. The use of both single-subject research designs and group research methods re-quiring inferential statistics have recently been repudiated (Ruck-deschel & Farris, 1981; Kagle, 1982; Cowger, 1985; Heineman, 1981). It is contended that objective knowledge of social work practice is impossible to obtain, and that the effort to obtain such information is a form of pseudoscience (Heineman-Peiper, 1985). Instead, we are told that we should adopt more qualitative methodologies, research strategies that have yet, to our knowl-edge, produce validated practice methods. We are puzzled by those who would have us abandon the accepted principles of scientific inquiry which have proven so useful to our profession and in every other area of human endeavor to which they have been applied. Certain limitations in the hypothetico-deductive approach to social work inquiry are widely recognized. For example, the difficulties in using single subject research designs cannot be minimized (Thomas, 1978) but the solution is to refine and expand these approaches, not to abandon them (Gambrill & Barth, 1981; Thyer & Curtis, 1983). The abuse of inferential statistics in group research is also common, but again the solution is the proper application of such methods, not their repudiation (Hudson, Thyer & Stocks, in press).

Heineman-Peiper (1985) has recently pointed out some potential inadequacies of the traditional methods of scientific inquiry, methods especially characteristic of behavioral social work. Her proposed solution is for social work to substitute approaches such as "ecology, phenomenology, ethonomethodology, structuralism, hermeneutics and functionalism "(Heineman-Peiper, 1985, p. 4). We believe that our profession is ill-served by those who disparage conventional scientific inquiry and advocate qualitative approaches at the expense of quantitative ones. We are just now beginning to see the fruits of several decades of conscientious practice research, efforts which are being repaid in the form of a developing body of empirical literature supportive of social work services. These favorable outcomes suggest the continued utility of adopting the highest standards of scientific rigor in our attempts to produce useful knowledge for social work practitioners, clients, students and scholars. It would seem that the ideal solution would be for the advocates of qualitative research to stop disparaging quantitative approaches and to set about the serious business of producing the practice knowledge which they claim will be forthcoming from their perspective. Our profession would be better served by publishing examples of clinically relevant qualitative research instead of continued perjorative statements on the inadequacy of quantitative approaches and of those who use them. We would see it as a strength to have a segment of our profession hard at work employing quantitative research strategies and another group vigorously producing qualitatively-derived knowledge.

As guest editors of this work, we were most fortunate to obtain, from some of the foremost authorities in the field of behavioral social work, contributions that represent a variety of substantive areas of practice. All share the common elements of being derived from contemporary learning theories, have an emphasis on high standards of scientific inquiry, and address serious problems of individual and social significance. We believe that this collection of articles describing empirically-based practice and quantitative research findings effectively illustrates the validity of these approaches to social work knowledge. The importance of " . . . an understanding and appreciation of the necessity of a scientific, analytic approach to knowledge building and practice" (Council on Social Work Education, 1982, p. 10) has been recognized in the current Curriculum Policy for BSW and MSW education. The work represents the vitality of this perspective. Four of the articles report original research findings that employ either conventional group research methods (Wodarski; Cheatham) or single-subject approaches to practice evaluation (Wong et al.; Pinkston). The other articles, contributed by leading scholars in their respective fields report comprehensive reviews of the state of the art in behavioral social work pertaining to selected substantive areas. A number of treatment modalities are described by our authors, including individual treatment (Steketee; Wong et al.; Levy; Pinkston), marital and family therapy (Polster et al.; Harrison; Thomas et al.), and group interventions (Gilchrist et al.; Wodarski). This diversity suggests the potential of behavioral social work as a comprehensive approach to practice at all levels (Thyer, 1987). The area of community-based interventions remains underdeveloped within the field of behavioral social work, although related disciplines are rapidly expanding their use of interventions derived from learning theory in the community arena.

The editors would like to express their gratitude to the contributors in producing this special work for their willing collaboration. The quality of their scholarship and their scientific integrity made editing these articles a rare intellectual pleasure.

Bruce A. Thyer
Walter W. Hudson

REFERENCES

Council on Social Work Education (1982). Curriculum policy for the Master's degree and Baccalaureate degree programs in social work education. *Social Work Education Reporter, 30*(3), 5-12.

Cowger, C. (1984). Statistical significance tests: Scientific ritualism or scientific method. *Social Service Review, 58*, 358-372.

Gambrill, E. D. & Barth, R. P. (1980). Single-case study designs revisited. *Social Work Research and Abstracts, 16*(3), 15-20.

Heineman, M. B. (1981). The obsolete scientific imperative in social work research. *Social Service Review, 55*, 371-397.

Heineman-Peiper, M. B. (1985). The future of social work research. *Social Work Research and Abstracts, 21*(4), 3-11.

Hudson, W. W., Thyer, B. A. & Stocks, J. T. (in press). Assessing the importance of experimental outcomes. *Journal of Social Service Research, 8,*87-98.

Kagle, J. D. (1982). Using single-subject measures in practice decisions: Systematic documentation or distortion? *Arete, 7*(2). 1-9.

Reid, W. J. & Hanrahan, P. (1982). Recent evaluations of social work: Grounds for optimism. *Social Work, 27*, 328-340.

Rubin, A. (1985). Practice effectiveness: More grounds for optimism. *Social Work, 30*, 469-476.

Ruckdeschel, R. & Farris, B. (1981). Assessing practice: A critical look at the single-case design. *Social Casework, 62*, 413-419.

Skinner, B. F. (1974). *About behaviorism.* New York: Knopf.

Thomas, E. J. (1978). Research and service in single-subject experimentation: Conflicts and choices. *Social Work Research and Abstracts, 14*(4), 20-31.

Thyer, B. A. (1981). Behavioral social work: A bibliography. *International Journal of Behavioral Social Work and Abstracts, 1*, 229-223.

Thyer, B. A. (1985). Textbooks in behavioral social work: A bibliography. *The Behavior Therapist, 8*, 161-162.

Thyer, B. A. (1987). Contingency analysis: Towards a unified theory for social work practice. *Social Work, 32*, 150-157.

Thyer, B. A. & Curtis, G. C. (1983). The repeated pretest-posttest single-subject experiment: A new design for empirical clinical practice. *Journal of Behavior Therapy and Experimental Psychiatry, 14*, 311-315.

Videka-Sherman, L. (1985). *Harriett M. Bartlett practice effectiveness project report to NASW board of directors.* New York: National Association of Social Workers.

Behavioral Treatment
of Chronic Psychiatric Patients

Stephen E. Wong
James E. Woolsey
Estrella Gallegos

SUMMARY. Behavioral treatments for hallucinations and delusions, aggressive and destructive responses, inappropriate social behavior, poor self-care and grooming, and deficient recreational and vocational skills in chronic psychiatric patients are reviewed. Consideration is given to the short-term, long-term, and generalized effects of these interventions. Three case studies illustrate behavioral procedures of consumable reinforcement, response cost, graphic feedback, differential reinforcement of other behavior (DRO), and overcorrection. The potential contribution of clinical social workers in applying such programs on a psychiatric unit is discussed.

This article reviews learning-based treatments for functional disorders manifested by chronic psychiatric patients. The population presents a formidable challenge for clinical social workers with a bewildering array of problem behaviors that are unaffected by conventional therapies. The efficacy of behavioral interventions for ameliorating these disorders has been well documented

---

Dr. Wong is Program Director and Mr. Woolsey is Unit Director of the Behavioral Treatment Unit, Northeast Florida State Hospital, Macclenny, Florida 32063. Ms. Gallegos is a clinical social worker at the Behavioral Rehabilitation Unit, Las Vegas Medical Center, P.O. Box 1388, Las Vegas, New Mexico 87701. The authors thank Miguel Larranaga, MA, who served as primary therapist on Case Study 1. Appreciation also goes to J. Pete Martinez, RN, Cecilia Archuleta, LPN, Jessie Archuleta, LPN, Maria Clayton, LPN, and the other staff of the Behavioral Rehabilitation Unit for their assistance in Case Study 2, and to the staff of the Clinical Research Unit, Camarillo State Hospital, for their help in Case Study 3. Reprint requests should be addressed to Dr. Wong.

7

(Liberman, Wallace, Teigen & Davis, 1974; Paul & Lentz, 1977: Wong, Massel, Mosk & Liberman, 1986); however, adoption of behavioral treatments in mental hospitals has not kept pace with research advances. This probably has been due to the medical establishment's providence over these facilities (Hersen & Bellack, 1978), and an unawareness of what the behavioral approach has to offer in the management of psychiatric disorders (Brady, 1973).

A sizable proportion of social workers — more than one-fifth of the National Association of Social Workers (Morris, 1974) — are employed in psychiatric settings. Although the behavioral social work literature is steadily expanding (Thyer, 1985), little has been written about psychiatric social work from a behavioral perspective. Existing articles have briefly described ward programs (Aveni, 1974; Stone & Nelson, 1979) or family-centered interventions with less severely disturbed clients (Hudson, 1975, 1976, 1978). More comprehensive review of treatments suitable for chronic, institutionalized mental patients is lacking. Given the profession's involvement in this field and the complex and refractory nature of psychiatric disorders, there is a need to become better acquainted with the full range of available behavioral techniques. This paper will examine learning-based interventions for a variety of dysfunctions in chronic psychiatric patients, and consider how social workers may aid in their implementation.

We will cover behavioral interventions to decrease hallucinatory and delusional speech, assaultive and destructive behavior, and bizarre stereotypies, as well as treatments to increase social skills, self-care and grooming, recreational activity, and vocational behavior. Case studies will exemplify some of the above therapeutic procedures. These case studies are drawn from the first author's work at the Behavioral Rehabilitation Unit of the Las Vegas Medical Center, Las Vegas, New Mexico, and the Clinical Research Unit of the Camarillo State Hospital, Camarillo, California. Both state facilities are locked psychiatric units designated for the treatment and management of chronic mental patients. A section preceding the conclusion will discuss generalization of therapy effects across settings and time.

HALLUCINATIONS AND DELUSIONS

Hallucinatory behaviors are verbal self-reports of idiosyncratic sensory experiences (e.g., complaints about hearing voices), or vocal or motor responses indicating that the subject perceives · something that doesn't exist (e.g., talking or gesturing into the empty air). Delusional behaviors are erroneous verbalizations or related actions (e.g., a patient claiming that he is Jesus Christ or that he is being persecuted) which persist in the face of overwhelming contradictory evidence. Hallucinatory and delusional behavior are considered to be principal symptoms of schizophrenia (American Psychiatric Association, 1980) and are often amenable to treatment by chemotherapy (Andreasen & Olsen, 1982; Davis & Gierl, 1984). Alternately, when viewed as maladaptive responses, these behaviors may also be treated by modifying the client's environment.

Reinforcement of Incompatible Behavior

Psychotic speech has been modified in chronic mental patients by prompting and reinforcing desirable verbal behavior. In one study positive reinforcement consisted only of therapist attention which was given or withdrawn depending on whether or not the patient's speech was appropriate (Moss & Liberman, 1975). In most of the research using this approach, however, social reinforcement for appropriate speech has been combined with some form of tangible reinforcement. Staff or therapist attention has been joined with contingent cigarettes (Ayllon & Haughton, 1964), coffee and snacks (Liberman, Teigen, Patterson & Baker, 1973), access to a preferred work activity (Anderson & Alpert, 1974), and token reinforcement (Patterson & Teigen, 1973; Wincze, Leitenberg & Agras, 1972) in programs correcting bizarre or inaccurate speech. A comparison of social versus token reinforcement has shown the latter to be more potent in reducing psychotic verbalizations (Meichenbaum, 1969). While tangible reinforcement has proven to be an effective procedure for changing psychotic verbal behavior, there are limitations to this approach. Certain patients do not consume and are unmotivated by the usual tangible reinforcers (cigarettes, coffee, snacks, etc.) and will not alter their speech to earn these rewards.

To illustrate a successful application of this technique, we now present a case study in which a patient's delusional speech was treated using reinforcement procedures. This client's verbalizations interfered with her placement planning, therefore, it was fitting that therapy be conducted by the unit social worker.

Case Study 1: Tammy K. Tammy was a 24-year old woman with a diagnosis of schizophrenia, paranoid type. Prior to her present commitment to the Las Vegas Medical Center, she had been hospitalized four times for mental breakdowns. Conduct in the community leading to rehospitalization included promiscuity, staying in bed all day, neglecting self-care and eating, and periodic aggression. With the exception of promiscuity, which was prevented by staff supervision, these problems continued in the hospital setting. Another of Tammy's difficulties involved her claims that she did not belong in the hospital. Tammy would say that her admitting psychiatrist had promised that she would be hospitalized for only two weeks. Tammy would repeat this claim and demand to be released, even after being told that she had been legally committed for 6 months and that her admitting psychiatrist was no longer responsible for her care.

Behavioral treatment of delusional speech consisted of consumable reinforcement for accurate speech combined with response cost for inaccurate speech. Therapy sessions, each 10-15 minutes long, were conducted in the social worker's office adjacent to the ward. Sessions were structured around a series of questions about the patient's condition, her progress in the unit program, unit rules, and criteria for discharge from the hospital. In baseline, the social worker gave the patient negative feedback for delusional statements (e.g., "No, that's wrong Tammy. You will not go home in two weeks.") and positive feedback For accurate statements (e.g., "Yes, that's right. You must stay out of bed"). In the treatment phase, Tammy received the above feedback plus she earned one cigarette for every five accurate statements made -- up to a maximum of two cigarettes per session. After being warned about her first delusional statement, she also lost one cigarette for every delusional statement emitted. Two weeks into training, the warning preceding cigarette loss was no longer given.

Results of this program are displayed in Figure 1. The upper

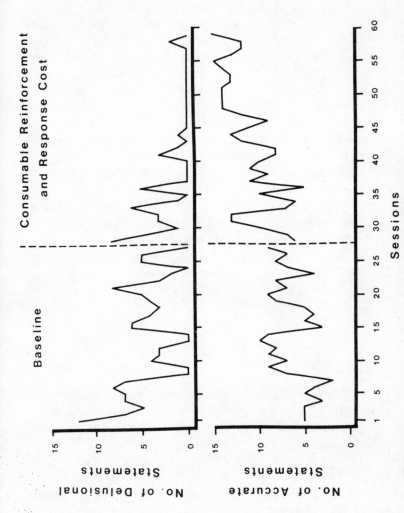

Figure 1. Data from Case Study 1. Upper graph shows the number of delusional statements and the lower graph the number of accurate statements emitted per session in baseline and treatment conditions.

11

graph depicts the number of delusional statements per session and the lower graph the number of accurate statements per session. During baseline, the number of delusional statements was highly variable and averaged 4.2; in the same period, a more consistent level of accurate statements was observed averaging 6.3. With the introduction of reinforcement and response cost procedures, the number of delusional statements gradually declined until by the 18th treatment session it fell to zero, where it stayed for all but one of the remaining sessions of the study. Concomitant changes were obtained in accurate speech, whose average level rose to 10.7 statements per session.

The cessation of delusional statements permitted the social worker and other professional staff to discuss Tammy's current ward behavior and placement plans with her in a rational manner. This was an important step in modifying Tammy's behavior pattern by presenting a set of rules and by making her responsible for adhering to those rules. Staying in bed and poor grooming continued to be problems on the ward, and these were subsequently modified with an individual behavioral contract and an occupational therapy assignment. After a month of compliance with her behavioral contract and satisfactory performance on her job assignment, Tammy was discharged to live with a sister residing out-of-state.

Stimulus Interference

Besides being controlled by consequent stimuli, hallucinatory and delusional behavior can be affected by antecedent and concurrent environmental stimuli. Several studies have demonstrated that self-reported hallucinations (Anderson & Alpert, 1974; Alford & Turner, 1976; Turner, Hersen & Bellack, 1977; Alford, Fleece & Rothblum, 1982) and overt motor behavior indicative of hallucinations (Alford et al., 1982) can be nearly eliminated by engaging subjects in conversation unrelated to their delusional beliefs. One experiment has shown that non-social stimuli in the form of a ringing bell suppressed hallucinatory self-talk in a schizophrenic patient (Turner et al., 1977). Two uncontrolled case reports also suggested that listening to the radio (Feder, 1982) and watching television (Magen, 1983) could have similar therapeutic effects in interrupting hallucinatory behavior. Related research has demonstrated that involvement in independent recreational activities can supplant self-talk and perseverative motoric behaviors in long-term institutionalized patients (Wong et al., 1984).

Punishment

Consequent stimuli that lower the probability of behavior can be programmed to weaken psychotic speech. In an early case study using punishment, a schizophrenic man was taught to self-administer a mild electric shock whenever he heard hallucinatory voices (Bucher & Fabricatore, 1970). Faradic shock has also been applied in two single-subject experiments during therapy sessions whenever patients reported auditory hallucinations (Alford & Turner, 1976; Turner et al., 1977). Observational data from one of the above experiments showed response suppression generalized to the ward environment, while anecdotal data from both investigations showed that auditory hallucinations remained at low levels on 6-month and 1-year follow-up assessments.

Timeout from reinforcement, in the form of confinement within a locked and barren room, has also been applied as an aversive consequence to decrease non-directed vocalizations occurring on the hospital ward. Self-talk and mumbling in a middle-aged chronic schizophrenic woman were reduced by one-half through the use of contingent locked timeout lasting 10 minutes (Haynes & Geddy, 1973). Hallucinatory and delusional verbalizations in another female schizophrenic were similarly suppressed when they were consequated with 15 minutes of locked timeout (Davis, Wallace, Liberman & Finch, 1976).

AGGRESSIVE AND DESTRUCTIVE BEHAVIOR

Most state civil commitment laws dictate that persons who are involuntarily confined in mental hospitals present a danger to themselves, or others, or be gravely disabled (American Bar Association, 1979). Because of these legal criteria, the most violent and low-functioning mentally disturbed persons are concentrated in the closed public institutions. Not surprisingly, aggressive and destructive acts are a frequent occurrence in these settings and pose a major clinical and administrative problem (Wong, Slama & Liberman, 1985). Viewing aggressive and destructive acts as behavioral excesses, learning-oriented treatments have attempted to reinforce alternate appropriate behavior as well as to directly weaken antagonistic responding.

Reinforcement of Incompatible Behavior

Aggressive and destructive behavior can be associated with inadequate social skills for satisfying one's needs or for resolving interpersonal conflicts. Social skills training is an attractive method for treating antagonistic behavior, because it employs only positive procedures and involves no aversive stimuli. Despite these advantages, it rarely has been utilized with chronic psychiatric patients. In an early application of this technique, a highly aggressive, brain-damaged patient was successfully treated with contingency contracts and assertiveness training (Wallace, Teigen, Liberman & Baker, 1973). Assertiveness training consisted of instructions and roleplaying in how to deal with frustrating institutional situations. Introduction of the treatment package was associated with a near cessation of aggressive incidents on the ward; but, since this was an uncontrolled case study, results could not be directly attributed to training. A controlled multiple-baseline experiment teaching social skills to two aggressive male inpatients better demonstrated the potential impact of this technique (Frederiksen, Jenkins, Foy & Eisler, 1976). Training increased appropriate requesting behaviors and decreased hostile behaviors in role-played situations, and also improved performance in contrived on-ward interactions used to assess generalization.

Punishment

Punishment of mental patient's aggressive and destructive behavior has generally been limited to the withdrawal of positive reinforcers or the application of mild aversive stimuli. While any sort of punishment of mental patients is entangled in legal and ethical controversy (Wexler, 1984), the empirical support for employing punishment procedures to reduce undesired behavior is voluminous and growing (Walters & Grusec, 1977; Harris & Ersner-Hershfield, 1978; Axelrod & Apsche, 1983; Matson & DiLorenzo, 1984). In theory myriad environmental stimuli could function as punishing events, but only a few punishment procedures have been applied and evaluated with chronic mental patients.

Seclusionary timeout from reinforcement, or confinement within a locked and barren room, is probably the most common behavioral intervention for severe aggressive, destructive, and disruptive behavior. Seclusionary timeout differs from traditional seclusion employed in psychiatric facilities along a number of lines: (1) the intervention is utilized as a planned treatment procedure rather than as a mere emergency measure; (2) the procedure is applied consistently after each occurrence of the target behavior; (3) the length of timeout is set at the minimum effective duration necessary to diminish future occurrences of the target behavior; and (4) data is used to substantiate that the treatment program is having its intended effect, and therefore, that the consequence is actually punishing the target response (Liberman & Wong, 1985).

Varying outcomes have been reported with different timeout durations and different groups of patients. Paul and Lentz (1977) found that 2-hour timeout intervals were ineffective and that lengthy 24-hour timeouts were needed to control aggression in their chronic back-ward patients with mixed psychiatric disorders. In contrast, work done by one of the present authors with a similarly chronic population has shown the potency of 15-60 minute timeouts for modifying a variety of assaultive and destructive behaviors (Wong et al., 1985). The latter finding is corroborated by data showing the effectiveness of brief 5-minute timeouts in eliminating disruptive and self-injurious behavior in chronic schizophrenic patients (Cayner & Kiland, 1974). Thus, under some circumstances, short periods of timeout from reinforcement can effectively decrease dangerous and destructive behavior.

Overcorrection is another potent technique for reducing antagonistic behavior in chronic mental patients. Four features distinguish overcorrection (Foxx & Azrin, 1972, 1973): (1) reeducation in desired prosocial responses (through explanation or engaging in the overcorrection exercise); (2) removal of reinforcement for the undesired behavior (e.g., return of stolen articles); (3) timeout from reinforcement (interruption of all other ongoing activities during overcorrection); and (4) an effortful task returning the problem situation to a state improved over that before the disturbance occurred (e.g., apologizing to offended parties and innocent bystanders, cleaning and repairing damaged and undamaged objects).

A pioneering study of overcorrection with chronic psychiatric patients involved four females with multiple diagnoses, who engaged in physical assault, verbal abuse, and property destruction (Sumner, Mueser, Hsu & Morales, 1974). The overcorrection procedure required patients to apologize for their offenses and to promise not to repeat these acts. Using a variant of overcorrection that resembled seclusionary timeout, other investigators decreased yelling and swearing in a schizophrenic man (Klinge, Thrasher, Myers, 1975). The intervention in this case study was 1-hour or more of required relaxation in bed for each disruptive outburst. Overcorrection has also been systematically compared to a DRI schedule (differential reinforcement of incompatible behavior; reinforcement given every hour for the absence of aggression) in a program reducing aggressive responses in an elderly schizophrenic woman (Matson & Stephens, 1977). The patient's aggressive behavior of throwing trash in other people's faces was virtually eliminated by requiring her to apologize to her victim and pick up trash for 5 minutes after every aggressive incident. By contrast, the DRI procedure had no influence on the frequency of aggression.

SOCIAL SKILLS

Many chronic psychiatric patients lack elementary verbal and non-verbal behaviors needed for interpersonal communication (Bellack & Hersen, 1978; Christoff & Kelly, 1985). Inadequacies of this sort impinge on all areas of functioning and diminish the likelihood of normal adjustment. Social skills training is a proven technique for teaching psychiatric patients variform interpersonal responses, such as: eye contact and facial expressions (Eisler, Blanchard, Fitts & Williams, 1978; Finch & Wallace, 1977; Hersen, Eisler & Miller, 1974); rudimentary greeting responses (Kale, Kale, Whelan & Hopkins, 1968); assertive behaviors (Frederiksen et al., 1976; Hersen & Bellack, 1976; Hersen, Turner, Edelstein & Pinkston, 1975); and conversational skills (Holmes, Hansen & St. Lawrence, 1984; Kelly, Urey & Patterson, 1980; Martinez-Diaz et al., 1983; Urey, Laughlin & Kelly, 1979).

Social skills training with chronic psychiatric patients has generally employed the standard format used with normal or minimally impaired individuals (see, for example: Schinke, Gilchrist, Smith & Wong, 1979). This treatment package consists of: (1) instructions describing and giving a rationale for the behavior being taught; (2) modeling or demonstration of the desired response; (3) rehearsal or practice of the target behavior; and (4) positive consequences (e.g., praise) for desired performances and negative consequences (e.g., corrective feedback) for faulty performances. Treatment usually occurs within the context of a series of role-played interactions enacted with a training confederate and supervised by a therapist.

Standard social skills training procedures are ill-adapted for regressed schizophrenic patients with severe attentional or memory dysfunctions. A stimulus control procedure that simplifies learning tasks has been designed for teaching social skills to this more seriously disabled subgroup (Liberman, Massel, Mosk & Wong, 1985). The stimulus control procedure teaches individual target responses—like the conversational question, "What did you do last night?"—within structured sessions that focus on discrete training trials. The procedure minimizes irrelevant stimuli, repeatedly trains target responses until they are mastered, and periodically reviews trained responses to ensure skill retention and to prevent confusion with new items. A controlled within-subject experiment has shown this format to be more potent than the standard approach for teaching withdrawn chronic schizophrenics the conversational skills of asking questions, giving compliments, making self-disclosures, and inviting someone to join in a mutual activity (Massel et al., 1984).

Although behavioral interventions to modify social response patterns have usually conceptualized clients' problems in terms of skills deficits, individuals may also have behavioral excesses in this area. The following paragraphs describe a case study in which social workers, psychologists, and nursing and attendant personnel joined together in applying a unit program to reduce highly disruptive social behavior in a mildly retarded woman.

Case Study 2: Priscilla B. Priscilla was a 37-year-old woman with a diagnosis of mild mental retardation and organic personality syndrome. She had a history of 15 prior hospitalizations to the Las Vegas Medical Center, and the present admission ensued after she was arrested for illegally entering a private home. On the hospital ward, Priscilla was utterly obnoxious and irritating to those near her. Her behavior consisted of incessant complaints, accusations, and demands, with tearful outbursts in which she would scream and cry. Actual disagreements with staff and or imagined offenses by others could trigger these emotional scenes. Priscilla would claim that staff and fellow patients were persecuting her, and say that her conflicts with other people would disappear if she were "not locked in the unit all day long."

The behavioral program for Priscilla centered around graphic feedback plus a response cost procedure in which inappropriate behavior resulted in a 24-hour loss of grounds privileges. Throughout baseline and treatment phases of the program, all unit staff who encountered her during the day recorded the frequency of inappropriate demanding, accusations, complaining, and emotional outbursts on a cumulative bar graph that was posted in the nursing station in a location visible to the client. Since Priscilla had asserted that all of her interpersonal problems would vanish once she was allowed to leave the ward during the day, she was first given grounds privileges on a non-contingent basis during a 9-day baseline period. In the subsequent treatment phase, a red criterion line was drawn on the graph; and, if the cumulative daily frequency of inappropriate behavior exceeded this criterion, Priscilla lost her grounds privileges for one day. The criterion level at which grounds privileges were contingently withdrawn was gradually lowered as treatment progressed.

Results of this ward program are displayed in Figure 2. Despite Priscilla's claims, during the 9-day baseline she continued to emit an average of 21 inappropriate behaviors per day, with a minimum of 9 inappropriate behaviors a day. Following institution of the criterion and contingency governing grounds privi-

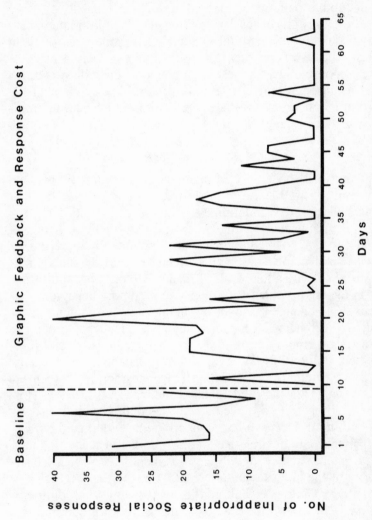

Figure 2. Data from Case Study 2. Graph displays the number of inappropriate social responses emitted daily in baseline and treatment conditions.

19

leges, Priscilla had her first day with no inappropriate behavior. Two days later another 24-hour period passed without a single inappropriate behavior being recorded. After this hiatus, Priscilla's disruptive pattern re-emerged at such an intensity that she lost all grounds privileges for a solid week. Inappropriate behavior then steadily declined until the end of the study. Throughout the last 10 days of treatment, Priscilla exhibited only 4 inappropriate responses. Due to these improvements Priscilla was transferred to an open unit whose staff continued to implement the above program. She was discharged from the hospital approximately 2 months later.

SELF-CARE AND GROOMING

The outward appearance of many chronic psychiatric patients is unkempt, dirty, bizarre, or abnormal in other ways. Deficiencies in self-care may undermine patients' social functioning, endanger their physical health, and stigmatize them as having a mental disorder. While clinicians have traditionally viewed poor self-care as a manifestation of patients' mental dysfunction, it may also be seen as the result of inadequate prompts and incentives in the environment for acceptable grooming behavior.

Seeking to change behavior by modifying environmental conditions, researchers have increased the frequency of grooming responses by employing reinforcement procedures. Social reinforcement in the form of stars posted for patients' achievements (Glickman, Plutchik & Landau, 1973), and food reinforcement in the form of the hospital lunch (Glickman et al., 1973; Hollander & Horner, 1975) have been made contingent on appropriate grooming in successful training programs with mixed psychiatric patients. Studies that have compared the efficacy of social reinforcement versus tangible reinforcement have shown the superiority of the latter technique with chronic patients (Glickman et al., 1973; Mertons & Fuller, 1963). Although food reinforcement has been shown to be a potent incentive for proper grooming, ethical considerations can make it unfeasible especially when it involves withholding patients' meals.

Token economy programs offer additional incentives over and above the essential requirements for institutional life, and have been frequently used to improve self-care behavior without denying patients their basic needs (Ayllon & Azrin, 1968; Liberman et al., 1974; Paul & Lentz, 1977). In these programs a certain number of tokens, exchangeable for a variety of back-up reinforcers, are given to patients depending on the quality of their appearance during inspection times. One evaluation of a token economy that focused solely on personal care behavior found a small but consistent positive effect of contingent tokens on daily grooming ratings (Lloyd & Garlington, 1968). Another analysis of token reinforcement showed that it could exert a strong impact when tied to a single self-care response – in this case, shoe cleaning (Winkler, 1970). In a more recent token economy program, grooming behaviors such as washing face, combing hair, shaving, brushing teeth, and dressing neatly were increased in psychiatric inpatients by prompting these responses with verbal instructions, modeled demonstrations, and posters describing the desired behaviors; and by reinforcing these behaviors with praise and tokens exchangeable for edibles, clothing items, and privileges (Nelson & Cone, 1979).

Not all self-care problems are suitable for treatment with prompting and token reinforcement. The following case study typifies how psychiatric patients exhibit unusual behaviors that elude ward programs and that require individualized treatment. The intervention in this study was a DRO schedule plus overcorrection to modify an obnoxious personal behavior in an extremely low-functioning chronic patient.

Case Study 3: Sammy M. Sammy was a 38-year-old, male chronic schizophrenic with a 20-year hospitalization history. On his transfer to the Clinical Research Unit at Camarillo State Hospital, the patient was very withdrawn and nearly mute, occasionally responding to questions with, "I donno." Contributing to Sammy's social isolation were offensive behaviors of frequently picking his nose in public, spitting, and smearing mucus and spittle on himself and nearby objects. Because of these behaviors, peers had ostracized the patient and had driven him to secluded areas of the ward where he spent much of the day lying on the floor.

Treatment of Sammy's undesirable behaviors consisted of differential reinforcement of other behavior (DRO) and overcorrection. The DRO schedule initially involved reinforcing the patient (giving him a cigarette) if he had not picked his nose, spit, or smeared in the preceding 30 minutes. The DRO interval was gradually lengthened until the patient had to refrain from the above inappropriate behaviors for 2 full hours before receiving reinforcement. A data sheet was posted in the nursing station containing DRO intervals for the entire day, and spaces to record the time of reinforcer delivery and responsible staff initials. The frequency of inappropriate behaviors was also recorded on this sheet, as it was observed by unit personnel on the ward. The overcorrection procedure required that immediately following each observed instance of nose-picking, spitting, or mucus smearing, the patient wash his hands or wipe the soiled clothing or object with a moist towel for 5 minutes. The patient would usually perform the overcorrection exercise with verbal prompts, but on rare occasions light manual guidance was required to have him complete the procedure. Sammy's behavior was so objectionable to nursing staff that the psychologist and social worker were unable to convince the former of the merits of collecting baseline data. Hence, in this case study treatment and data collection were initiated simultaneously.

Results of the individual program are displayed in Figure 3. In the first and second weeks on the ward, the patient's average daily frequency of spitting and mucus smearing was 37 and 29.6, respectively. By the seventh week of treatment the average daily frequency of these behaviors had fallen to 8.4. During the subsequent 7 months, the target behaviors were reduced even further. The average daily frequency of spitting and mucus smearing for the last two weeks of treatment was 2 and 0.6. Concomitant with this reduction in undesired behavior was increased acceptance by peers and unit personnel. Sammy no longer remained only in isolated parts of the unit, but began to mingle freely and became a "favorite" of many staff. Substantial improvements were noted in the quality and frequency of Sammy's interactions with other people on the ward.

RECREATIONAL BEHAVIOR

Like some elderly (McClannahan & Risley, 1974) and many retarded persons (Matson & Marchetti, 1980), chronic mental patients often fail to engage in productive and socially acceptable

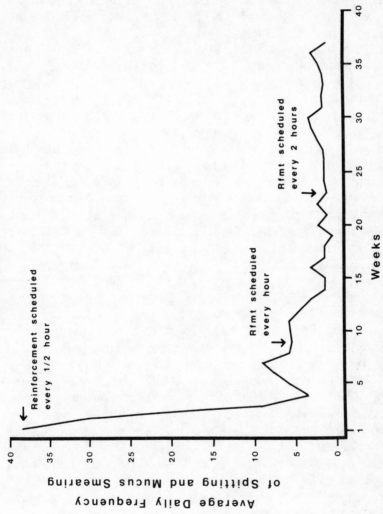

Figure 3. Data from Case Study 3. Graph displays the average daily frequency of spitting and mucus smearing during treatment with a DRO schedule and overcorrection.

leisure-time activities. Deficient recreational skills mean the loss of reinforcement associated with these activities as well as diminished opportunity for social interaction. Without appropriate diversions to fill the waking hours, individuals may also experience depression or become engrossed in maladaptive self-stimulatory behaviors (Ferster, 1973).

Improving recreational skills and raising activity levels in chronic mental patients is a goal that has been generally overlooked by behavioral researchers. Two notable exceptions to this trend were studies applying contingency management to increase exercise behavior. In the first study, which was an evaluation of a comprehensive token economy program, token reinforcement and scheduled exercise sessions were employed to increase physical activity of patients in a locked psychiatric ward (Nelson & Cone, 1979). In the second study, consumable reinforcement was utilized to encourage workouts on an exercise bicycle by two former mental patients in group home (Thyer, Irvine & Santa, 1984). Both studies increased the amount of subjects' daily exercise, presumably promoting their physical fitness and health.

Sedentary forms of activity and recreational therapy are commonplace in psychiatric settings, but scant objective data exists to validate their therapeutic advantages. Recently, however, social workers have collaborated with recreational therapists in research revealing positive effects of recreational activities on bizarre stereotypies in chronic psychiatric patients. In a series of single-case experiments carried out at the Clinical Research Unit at Camarillo State Hospital, supervised group activities (consisting of art projects, table games, and discussion groups) were shown to eliminate low-rate obsessive-compulsive ruminating in one patient and grotesque posturing in a second, as well as greatly reduce high-rate mumbling in a third individual (Wong, Terranova, Marshall, Banzett & Liberman, 1982). Subsequent experiments further demonstrated that mumbling and self-talk in two schizophrenic patients were substantially lessened during engagement in unsupervised, independent recreational activities of magazine reading and model building (Wong, Terranova, Marshall, Banzett & Liberman, 1983). A generalization assessment disclosed that response replacement was limited to the time periods in which activities were present; thus, maximum benefits from recreational interventions would be obtained by scheduling them regularly throughout the clients' day. The therapeutic effects of structured activities also have been documented with groups of patients and alternate observational measures. In a study employing the Time-Sample Behavior Checklist (Paul & Lentz, 1977), a comprehensive observational code, recreational and housework-like activities were shown to reduce numerous inappropriate "crazy" behaviors by approximately 70% in nine schizophrenic patients. Perhaps more importantly, structured activities increased the amount of appropriate "concurrent" behaviors exhibited by these individuals almost five times over the baseline level (Wong et al., 1984). The above investigations have begun to quantify recreational therapy's clinical impact in replacing psychotic behaviors and in evoking appropriate and productive behavior that would not otherwise occur.

VOCATIONAL SKILLS

Work is central to human life and therefore is an essential aspect of psychiatric rehabilitation (Strauss & Carpenter, 1974; Strauss, Glazer, Geller & Hafez, 1981). The demands of work in modern society accentuate the handicaps of chronic mental patients and their failings in this area are conspicuous. Unemployment has been found to be as high as 70% in the chronic mentally disabled (Goldstrom & Manderscheid, 1982). Employment rates following hospital discharge range between 10% to 30%, and only approximately 15% sustain their employment 1 to 5 years following discharge (Anthony, Buell, Sharratt & Althoff, 1972). These data attest to the importance of assisting psychiatric patients in preparing for, securing, and maintaining gainful employment.

Work experience contributing to rehabilitation can be provided for patients in the hospital setting. Utilizing a token economy program, chronic back-ward patients have been motivated to perform a multitude of clerical and custodial jobs (Ayllon & Azrin, 1965). Through procedures of prompting and shaping, responses to simple instructions can be gradually developed into sustained and productive labor by reinforcing successive approximations to the terminal goal (Ayllon & Azrin, 1968). A psychotic patient might initially be rewarded for merely complying with the request, "Please sit at this work bench," then for working 1 minute at a simple task, later for working 5 minutes continuously, and so on, until the patient could remain at a task lasting several hours. Therapists can employ these techniques to begin to restore adaptive functioning in even the most severely disturbed and deteriorated patients.

Behavioral training in job interviewing is another promising realm of vocational rehabilitation. Two studies have validated techniques for teaching job interviewing skills to psychiatric patients, one using an individual training format (Furman, Geller, Simon & Kelly, 1979), and the other a group format (Kelly, Laughlin, Claiborne & Patterson, 1979). In both studies, patients' performances in baseline and treatment phases were assessed in scripted, role-played interviews that were videotaped, and subsequently rated. Instruction focused on specific skill components such as providing positive information about previous work experiences and education, asking questions, gesturing, and expressing enthusiasm. Training consisted of exposure to videotaped models, behavioral rehearsal during simulated interviews, praise for appropriate responses and corrective feedback for inappropriate responses, coaching to improve performance, and the repetition of these steps. Combinations of the aforementioned procedures used in these two studies produced increases in skill components for all subjects, and gains for most subjects in pre- to post-treatment ratings obtained from an actual personnel manager.

Another step in vocational rehabilitation surrounds the problem of finding suitable job openings and effectively applying for available positions. Azrin and his associates (Azrin & Besalel, 1980; Azrin, Flores & Kaplan, 1975) have developed a "job-finding club" which produces a 70% to 80% employment rate in normal subjects. Their job club is an intensive and practical program involving: a systematic job search; use of social support groups; training in job interviewing, proper dress and grooming, and resume preparation; and careful follow-up on all job leads. A modified job club program developed for chronic mental patients at the Veterans Administration Medical Center at Brentwood, California, has produced comparable results with this special population (Jacobs, Kardashian, Kreinbring, Ponder & Simpson, 1984). The V.A. job club curriculum was divided into two parts: development of job finding and community survival skills. The latter set of skills included personal goal setting, problem solving, coping with daily problems, and maintaining one's employment. Skills were taught through lecture, programmed reading materials, roleplaying, and in-vivo exercises. Outcome data from the V.A. job club showed that 76% of the participants found jobs or entered full-time vocational training by the end of the program. Furthermore, as many as 67% remained employed after 6 months.

GENERALIZATION AND MAINTENANCE

Generalization is the carry-over of behavior change across stimulus conditions (e.g., physical and social environments) and across responses (e.g., to untreated behaviors). Maintenance is a special case of generalization referring to the carry-over of behavior change across time. Both generalization and maintenance are important factors in evaluating the significance of clinical interventions. Although few of the studies reviewed here thoroughly assessed both generalization and maintenance, we will summarize what is known about carry-over effects of the prior behavioral treatments.

Research on generalization indicates that the better the therapy situation prepares the client for the demands of the natural setting and the more it resembles the latter, the greater the likelihood of positive carry-over (Stokes & Baer, 1977). This axiom also applies to the previously discussed behavioral interventions with chronic psychiatric patients. Social skills training, which usually involves instruction within a series of different roleplays, has produced good generalization in novel role-played situations (Bellack et al., 1976; Eisler et al., 1978; Goldsmith & McFall, 1975; Hersen et al., 1975). However, this treatment mode has yielded poor generalization to extra-therapy settings (Gutride,

Goldstein, Hunter, 1973; Jaffe & Carlson, 1976; Shepherd, 1977), perhaps due to the easy discriminability of therapy sessions and the fact that training never occurs in-vivo. Yet transfer of learning can be facilitated by intermixing or reducing the difference between therapy and extra-therapy situations. For example, carry-over of recently trained social skills has been actuated by providing intermittent verbal prompts and reinforcement for trained responses in the setting where the target behavior is desired (Martinez-Diaz et al., 1983).

Extent of generalization also varies depending on the behavior being treated. Psychotic self-talk can be decelerated with several behavioral procedures; however, this response is resilient and often recovers its original operant level as treatment conditions are withdrawn (Haynes & Geddy, 1973; Wong et al., 1983), even if the withdrawal is gradual (Davis et al., 1976). Fortunately, a behavior rebounding in this manner is unusual, and this may be an outgrowth of self-talk having special self-stimulatory properties for certain individuals.

When treatment occurs in the situation where behavior change is desired, the issue of generalization diminishes. Hospital programs aimed at managing aggression and improving self-care have lessened the problem of obtaining generalization by modifying target behaviors on the ward where they occur. Timeout from reinforcement (Wong et al., 1985) and overcorrection (Matson & Stephens, 1977; Sumner et al., 1974) can be relied upon to control aggression in the hospital for many weeks or months, or for as long as treatment is continued. One study of a token economy has shown that gains in personal neatness were maintained even after the discontinuation of contingent token reinforcement (Elliott, Barlow, Hooper & Kingerlee, 1979). Of course, all of these programs were directed at behavior in the institution, and the absence of data on patients after they leave the hospital makes it difficult to know if newly taught behavior patterns generalize to community life. One program reviewed earlier which overcame the problem of generalization was the V.A. job-seeking club (Jacobs et al., 1984). This program assisted clients in the pursuit of employment in the real world, a locus of treatment that might be odd for other mental health professionals but quite familiar and comfortable for social workers.

While few behavioral programs for chronic mental patients have demonstrated broad and lasting changes after the removal of therapeutic contingencies, these interventions have often been judged by a double standard that overlooks similar weakness in prevailing biological treatments. It is widely accepted that antipsychotic medication, the dominant therapy for psychiatric disorders and the main competitor to behavioral treatment, helps to prevent relapse (Davis, Gosenfeld & Tsai, 1976) as long as patients adhere to their medication regimen. Medication compliance, however, is an serious problem prevalent in both psychiatric and non-psychiatric patients (Battle, Halliburton & Wallston, 1982). Furthermore, a relationship between the unpleasant side-effects of antipsychotic medication and noncompliance is beginning to be appreciated by psychiatrists (Van Putten, May & Marder, 1984). Thus, all existing treatments for chronic mental disorders are imperfect and deserve more empirical study to extend their boundaries of usefulness.

CONCLUSION

We have reviewed techniques derived from learning theory for modifying a variety of behavioral excesses and deficits in chronic psychiatric patients. Outcome research has validated the efficacy of the prior behavioral treatments for altering targeted responses. Three case studies illustrated how these procedures could be implemented on a psychiatric ward with a social worker as the primary therapist or as a member of an interdisciplinary treatment team.

Given psychiatry's minimal and unsteady support of behavioral research, the previous achievements are probably greater than what might be reasonable to expect of an immature technology in a foreign territory. While data shows that even the most severely disturbed patients are responsive to environmental stimuli and reinforcement contingencies, practical programs for modifying clients' behavior in institutions and in the community need further development and refinement. Prior work with this population consists mainly of exploratory studies or short-lived demonstration projects aimed at limited behavior change.

The role of a clinical social worker presented here was that of a member of an interdisciplinary treatment team. The multiplicity of professions joining together in the psychiatric setting requires an interdisciplinary approach, and the need for consistency in applying treatment contingencies demands that unit personnel operate as a team. If the person on the clinical team with the most behavioral expertise happens to be a social worker, then he or she should assume responsibility for developing, evaluating, and upgrading the unit program. This makes sense on a locked psychiatric ward (Marshall, Banzett, Kuehnel & Moore, 1983) or in an open community-based agency (Wodarski, 1976). By becoming proficient in behavioral technology, social workers can expand beyond the discharge planner role and provide needed leadership in the application of a powerful and under-utilized treatment modality.

REFERENCES

Alford, G. S., Fleece, L. & Rothblum, E. (1982). Hallucinatory-delusional verbalizations: Modification in a chronic schizophrenic by self-control and cognitive restructuring. *Behavior Modification, 6*, 421-435.

Alford, G. S. & Turner, S. M. (1976). Stimulus interference and conditioned inhibition of auditory hallucinations. *Journal of Behavior Therapy and Experimental Psychiatry, 7*, 155-160.

American Bar Association (1979). State laws governing civil commitment. In P. R. Friedman (Chair), *Legal rights of mentally disabled persons*, Vol. 1. Washington, DC: Practising Law Institute. (Reprinted from *Mental Disability Law Reporter*, 1979, *205*, 237-254.)

American Psychiatric Association (1980). *Diagnostic and statistical manual of mental disorders*. 3rd ed.; Washington, DC: American Psychiatric Association.

Anderson, L. T. & Alpert, M. (1974). Operant analysis of hallucination frequency in a hospitalized schizophrenic. *Journal of Behavior Therapy and Experimental Psychiatry, 5*, 13-18.

Andreasen, N. C. & Olsen, S. (1982). Negative vs. positive schizophrenia: Definition and validation. *Archives of General Psychiatry, 39*, 789-794.

Anthony, W. A., Buell, G. J., Sharratt, S. & Althoff, M. E. (1972). Efficacy of psychiatric rehabilitation. *Psychological Bulletin, 78*, 447-456.

Aveni, C. A. (1974). A behavior therapy program on a psychiatric ward. *Social Work, 19*, 136-138.

Axelrod, S. & Apsche, J. (Eds.) (1983). *The effects of punishment on human behavior*. New York: Academic Press.

Ayllon, T. & Azrin, N. H. (1965). The measurement and reinforcement of behavior of psychotics. *Journal of the Experimental Analysis of Behavior, 8*, 357-383.

Ayllon, T. & Azrin, N. (1968). *The token economy: A motivational system for therapy and rehabilitation.* Englewood Cliffs, NJ: Prentice-Hall.

Ayllon, T. & Haughton, E. (1964). Modification of symptomatic verbal behaviour of mental patients. *Behaviour Research and Therapy, 2,* 87-97.

Azrin, N. H. & Besalel, V. A. (1980). *Job-club counselors manual: A behavioral approach to vocational counseling.* Baltimore: University Park Press.

Azrin, N. H., Flores, T. & Kaplan, S. J. (1975). Job-finding club: A group-assisted program for obtaining employment. *Behaviour Research and Therapy, 13,* 17-27.

Battle, E. H., Halliburton, A. & Wallston, K. A. (1982). Self medication among psychiatric patients and adherence after discharge. *Journal of Psychosocial Nursing and Mental Health Services, 20,* 21-28.

Bellack, A. S. & Hersen, M. (1978). Chronic psychiatric patients: Social skills training. In M. Hersen & A. S. Bellack (Eds.), *Behavior therapy in the psychiatric setting.* Baltimore: Williams & Wilkins.

Bellack, A. S., Hersen, M. & Turner, S. M.. (1976). Generalization effects of social skills training in chronic schizophrenics: An experimental analysis. *Behaviour Research and Therapy, 14,* 391-398.

Brady, J. P. (1973). The place of behavior therapy in medical student and psychiatric resident training. *Journal of Nervous and Mental Disease, 157,* 21-26.

Bucher, B. & Fabricatore, J. (1970). Use of patient-administered shock to suppress hallucinations. *Behavior Therapy, 1,* 382-385.

Cayner, J. J. & Kiland, J. R. (1974). Use of brief time out with three schizophrenic patients. *Journal of Behavior Therapy and Experimental Psychiatry, 5,* 141-145.

Christoff, K. A. & Kelly, J. A. (1985). Social skills training with psychiatric patients. In M. A. Milan & L. L'Abata (Eds.), *Handbook of social skills training.* New York: Wiley.

Davis, J. M. & Gierl, B. (1984). Pharmacological treatment in the care of schizophrenic patients. In A. S. Bellack (Ed.), *Schizophrenia: Treatment, management, and rehabilitation.* Orlando, FL: Grune & Stratton, Inc.

Davis, J. M., Gosenfeld, L. & Tsai, C. C. (1976). Maintenance antipsychotic drugs do prevent relapse: A reply to Tobias and MacDonald. *Psychological Bulletin, 83,* 431-447.

Davis, J. R., Wallace, C. J., Liberman, R. P. & Finch, B. E. (1976). The use of brief isolation to suppress delusional and hallucinatory speech. *Journal of Behavior Therapy and Experimental Psychiatry, 7,* 269-275.

Eisler, R. M., Blanchard, E. B., Fitts, H. & Williams, J. G. (1978). Social skill training with and without modeling for schizophrenic and non-psychotic hospitalized psychiatric patients. *Behavior Modification, 2,* 147-172.

Elliott, P. A., Barlow, F., Hooper, A. & Kingerlee, P. E. (1979). Maintaining patients' improvements in a token economy. *Behaviour Research and Therapy, 17,* 355-367.

Feder, R. (1982). Auditory hallucinations treated by radio headphones. *American Journal of Psychiatry, 139,* 1188-1190.

Ferster, C. B. (1973). A functional analysis of depression. *American Psychologist, 28,* 857-870

Finch, B. E. & Wallace, C. J. (1977). Successful interpersonal skills training with schizophrenic inpatients. *Journal of Consulting and Clinical Psychology, 45,* 885-890.

Foxx, R. M. & Azrin, N. H. (1973). The elimination of autistic self-stimulatory behavior by overcorrection. *Journal of Applied Behavior Analysis, 6,* 1-14.

Foxx, R. M. & Azrin, N. H. (1972). Restitution: A method of eliminating aggressive-disruptive behavior of retarded and brain damaged patients. *Behaviour Research and Therapy, 10*, 15-27.

Frederiksen, L. W., Jenkins, J. O., Foy, D. W. & Eisler, R. M. (1976). Social skills training to modify abusive verbal outbursts in adults. *Journal of Applied Behavior Analysis, 9*, 117-125.

Furman, W., Geller, M., Simon, S. J. & Kelly, J. A. (1979). The use of a behavioral rehearsal procedure for teaching job-interviewing skills to psychiatric patients. *Behavior Therapy, 10*, 157-167.

Glickman, H., Plutchik, R. & Landau, H. (1973). Social and biological reinforcement in an open psychiatric ward. *Journal of Behavior Therapy and Experimental Psychiatry, 4*, 121-124.

Goldsmith, J. B. & McFall, R. M. (1975). Development and evaluation of an interpersonal skill-training program for psychiatric patients. *Journal of Abnormal Psychology, 84*, 51-58.

Goldstrom, I. & Manderscheid, R. (1982). The chronically mentally ill: A descriptive analysis from the uniform Client Data Instrument. *Community Support Services Journal, 2*, 4-9.

Gutride, M. E., Goldstein, A. P. & Hunter, G. F. (1973). The use of modeling and role playing to increase social interaction among asocial psychiatric patients. *Journal of Consulting and Clinical Psychology, 40*, 408-415.

Harris, S. L. & Ersner-Hershfield, R. (1978). Behavioral suppression of seriously disruptive behavior in psychotic and retarded patients: A review of punishment and its alternatives. *Psychological Bulletin, 85*, 1352-1375.

Haynes, S. N. & Geddy, P. (1973). Suppression of psychotic hallucinations through time-out. *Behavior Therapy, 4*, 123-127.

Hersen, M. & Bellack, A. S. (1976). A multiple-baseline analysis of social-skills training in chronic schizophrenics. *Journal of Applied Behavior Analysis, 9*, 239-245.

Hersen, M. & Bellack, A. S. (1978). Staff training and consultation. In M. Hersen & A. S. Bellack (Eds.), *Behavior therapy in the psychiatric setting*. Baltimore: Williams & Wilkins Company.

Hersen, M., Eisler, R. M. & Miller, P. M. (1974). An experimental analysis of generalization in assertive training. *Behaviour Research and Therapy, 12*, 295-310.

Hersen, M., Turner, S. M., Edelstein, B. A. & Pinkston, S. G. (1975). Effects of phenothiazines and social skills training in a withdrawn schizophrenic. *Journal of Clinical Psychology, 34*, 588-594.

Hollander, M. & Horner, V. (1975). Using environmental assessment and operant procedures to build integrated behaviors in schizophrenics. *Journal of Behavior Therapy and Experimental Psychiatry, 6*, 289-294.

Holmes, M. R., Hansen, D. J. & St. Lawrence, J. S. (1984). Conversational skills training with aftercare patients in the community: Social validation and generalization. *Behavior Therapy, 15*, 84-100.

Hudson, B. L. (1975). A behaviour modification project with chronic schizophrenics in the community. *Behaviour Research and Therapy, 13*, 239-341.

Hudson, B. L. (1976). Behavioural social work in a community psychiatric service. In M. R. Olsen (Ed.), *Differential approaches in social work with the mentally disordered*. Birmingham, UK: British Association of Social Workers.

Hudson, B. L. (1978). Behavioural social work with schizophrenic patients in the community. *British Journal of Social Work, 8*, 159-170.

Jacobs, H. E., Kardashian, S., Kreinbring, R. K., Ponder, R. & Simpson, A. R. (1984). A skills-oriented model for facilitating employment among psychiatrically disabled persons. *Rehabilitation Counseling Bulletin, 28*, 87-96.

Jaffe, P. G. & Carlson, P. M. (1976). Relative efficacy of modeling and instructions in eliciting social behavior from chronic psychiatric patients. *Journal of Consulting and Clinical Psychology, 44,* 200-207.

Kale, R. J., Kale, J. H., Whelan, P. A. & Hopkins, B. L. (1968). The effects of reinforcement on the modification, maintenance, and generalization of social responses of mental patients. *Journal of Applied Behavior Analysis, 1,* 307-314.

Kelly, J. A., Laughlin, C., Claiborne, M. & Patterson, J. (1979). A group procedure for teaching job interviewing skills to formerly hospitalized psychiatric patients. *Behavior Therapy, 10,* 299-310.

Kelly, J. A., Urey, J. R. & Patterson, J. T. (1980). Improving heterosocial conversational skills of male psychiatric patients through a small group training procedure. *Behavior Therapy, 11,* 179-183.

Klinge, V., Thrasher, P. & Myers, S. (1975). Use of bed-rest overcorrection in a chronic schizophrenic. *Journal of Behavior Therapy and Experimental Psychiatry, 6,* 69-73.

Liberman, R. P., Massel, H. K., Mosk, M. D. & Wong, S. E. (1985). Social skills training for chronic mental patients. *Hospital and Community Psychiatry, 36,* 396-403.

Liberman, R. P., Teigen, J., Patterson, R. & Baker, V. (1973). Reducing delusional speech in chronic paranoid schizophrenics. *Journal of Applied Behavior Analysis, 6,* 57-64.

Liberman, R. P., Wallace, C., Teigen, J. & Davis, J. (1974). Interventions with psychotic behaviors. In K. S. Calhoun, H. E. Adams & K. M. Mitchell (Eds.), *Innovative treatment methods in psychopathology.* New York: John Wiley & Sons, Inc.

Liberman, R. P. & Wong, S. E. (1985). Behavior analysis and therapy and restrictive procedures. In K. Tardiff (Chair), *Seclusion and restraint: The psychiatric uses.* Report of the American Psychiatric Association Task Force on the Psychiatric Uses of Seclusion and Restraint. Washington, DC: American Psychiatric Association.

Lloyd, K. E. & Garlington, W. K. (1968). Weekly variations in performance on a token economy psychiatric ward. *Behaviour Research and Therapy, 6,* 407-410.

Magen, J. (1983). Increasing external stimuli to ameliorate hallucinations. *American Journal of Psychiatry, 140,* 269-270.

Martinez-Diaz, J. A., Massel, H. K., Wong, S. E., Wiegand, W., Bowen, L., Edelstein, B. A., Marshall, B. D. & Liberman, R. P. (1983, December). Training and generalization of conversational skills in chronic schizophrenics. Paper presented at the World Congress of Behavior Therapy, Washington, DC.

Marshall, B. D., Banzett, L., Kuehnel, T. & Moore, J. (1983). Maintaining nursing staff performance on an intensive behavior therapy unit. *Analysis and Intervention in Developmental Disabilities, 3,* 193-204.

Massel, H. K., Bowen, L., Mosk, M. D., Wong, S. E., Zarate, R., Milan, M. A., Marshall, B. D. & Liberman, R. P. (1984, November). Conversational skills training for chronic psychiatric patients. Paper presented at the 18th Annual Convention of the Association for Advancement of Behavior Therapy, Philadelphia, PA.

Matson, J. L. & DiLorenzo, T. M. (1984). *Punishment and its alternatives: A new perspective for behavior modification.* New York: Springer Publishing Co.

Matson, J. L. & Marchetti, A. (1980). A comparison of leisure skills training procedures for the mentally retarded. *Applied Research in Mental Retardation, 1,* 113-122.

Matson, J. L. & Stephens, R. M. (1977). Overcorrection of aggressive behavior in a chronic psychiatric patient. *Behavior Modification, 1,* 559-564.

McClannahan, L. E. & Risley, T. R. (1974). Activities and materials for severely disabled geriatric patients. *Nursing Homes, 24*, 10-13.

Meichenbaum, D. H. (1969). The effects of instructions and reinforcement on thinking and language behavior of schizophrenics. *Behaviour Research and Therapy, 7*, 101-114.

Mertons, G. C. & Fuller, G. B. (1963). Conditioning of molar behavior in "regressed" psychotics. *Journal of Clinical Psychology, 19*, 333-337.

Morris, R. (1974). The place of social work in the human services. *Social Work, 19*, 519-531.

Moss, G. R. & Liberman, R. P. (1975). Empiricism in psychotherapy: Behavioural specification and measurement. *British Journal of Psychiatry, 126*, 73-80.

Nelson, G. L. & Cone, J. D. (1979). Multiple-baseline analysis of a token economy for psychiatric inpatients. *Journal of Applied Behavior Analysis, 12*, 255-271.

Patterson, R. L. & Teigen, J. R. (1973). Conditioning and post-hospital generalization of nondelusional responses in a chronic psychotic patient. *Journal of Applied Behavior Analysis, 6*, 65-70.

Paul, G. L. & Lentz, R. J. (1977). *Psychosocial treatment of chronic mental patients.* Cambridge, MA: Harvard University Press.

Schinke, S. P., Gilchrist, L. D., Smith, T. E. & Wong, S. E. (1979). Group interpersonal skills training in a natural setting: An experimental study. *Behaviour Research and Therapy, 17*, 149-154.

Shepherd, G. (1977). Social skills training: The generalization problem. *Behavior Therapy, 8*, 1008-1009.

Stone, M. E. & Nelson, G. L. (1979). Coordinated treatment for long-term psychiatric inpatients. *Social Work, 24*, 406-410.

Stokes, T. F. & Baer, D. M. (1977). An implicit technology of generalization. *Journal of Applied Behavior Analysis, 10*, 349-367.

Strauss, J. S. & Carpenter, W. T. (1974). The prediction of outcome in schizophrenia. *Archives of General Psychiatry, 31*, 37-42.

Strauss, J. S., Glazer, W., Geller, E. & Hafez, H. (1981). The role of work in recovery from schizophrenia. Paper presented at the meeting of the American Psychiatric Association, New Orleans, LA.

Sumner, J. H., Mueser, S. T., Hsu, L. & Morales, R. G. (1974). Overcorrection treatment for radical reduction of aggressive-disruptive behavior in institutionalized mental patients. *Psychological Reports, 35*, 655-662.

Thyer, B. A. (1985). Textbooks in behavioral social work: A bibliography. *The Behavior Therapist, 8*, 161-162.

Thyer, B. A., Irvine, S. & Santa, C. A. (1984). Contingency management of exercise by chronic schizophrenics. *Perceptual and Motor Skills, 58*, 419-425.

Turner, S. M., Hersen, M. & Bellack, A. S. (1977). Effects of social disruption. stimulus interference, and aversive conditioning on auditory hallucinations. *Behavior Modification, 1*, 249-258.

Urey, J. R., Laughlin, C. & Kelly, J. A. (1979). Teaching heterosocial conversational skills to male psychiatric inpatients. *Journal of Behavior Therapy and Experimental Psychiatry, 10*, 323-328.

Van Putten, T., May, P. R. A. & Marder, S. R. (1984). Response to antipsychotic medication: The doctor's and the consumer's view. *American Journal of Psychiatry, 141*, 16-19.

Wallace, C. J., Teigen, J. R., Liberman, R. P. & Baker, V. (1973). Destructive behavior treated by contingency contracts and assertive training: A case study. *Journal of Behavior Therapy and Experimental Psychiatry, 4*, 273-274.

Walters, G. C. & Grusec, J. E. (1977). *Punishment*. San Francisco: W. H. Freeman and Company.

Wexler, D. B. (1984). Legal aspects of seclusion and restraint. In K. Tardiff (Ed.), *The psychiatric uses of seclusion and restraint*. Washington, DC: American Psychiatric Press.

Wincze, J. P., Leitenberg, H. & Agras, W. S. (1972). The effects of token reinforcement and feedback on the delusional verbal behavior of chronic paranoid schizophrenics. *Journal of Applied Behavior Analysis, 5*, 247-262.

Winkler, R. C. (1970). Management of chronic psychiatric patients by a token reinforcement system. *Journal of Applied Behavior Analysis, 3*, 47-55.

Wodarski, J. S. (1976). Procedural steps in the implementation of behavior modification programs in open settings. *Journal of Behavior Therapy and Experimental Psychiatry, 7*, 133-136.

Wong, S. E., Massel, H. K., Mosk, M. D. & Liberman, R. P. (1986). Behavioral approaches to the treatment of schizophrenia. In G. D. Burrows, T. R. Norman & G. Rubinstein (Eds.), *Handbook of studies on schizophrenia, Part 2: Management and research*. Amsterdam, The Netherlands: Elsevier Science Publishers.

Wong, S. E., Slama, K. M. & Liberman, R. P. (1985). Behavioral analysis and therapy for aggressive psychiatric and developmentally disabled patients. In L. H. Roth (Ed.), *Clinical treatment of the violent person* (NIMH Monograph). Washington, DC: U.S. Government Printing Office.

Wong, S. E., Stewart, J., Terranova, M. D., Bowen, L., Zarate, R. & Zarate, R. (1984, May). Replacement of "crazy behavior" in psychiatric patients during structured activities. Paper presented at the 10th Annual Convention of the Association for Behavior Analysis, Nashville. TN.

Wong, S. E., Terranova, M. D., Marshall, B. D., Banzett, L. K. & Liberman, R. P. (1982, November). Reduction of bizarre stereotypic behavior in chronic psychiatric patients during recreational activities. Paper presented at the 16th Annual Convention of the Association for Advancement of Behavior Therapy, Los Angeles, CA.

Wong, S. E., Terranova, M. D., Marshall, B. D., Banzett, L. K. & Liberman, R. P. (1983, May). Reducing bizarre stereotypic behavior in chronic psychiatric patients: Effects of supervised and independent recreational activities. Paper presented at the 9th Annual Convention of the Association for Behavior Analysis. Milwaukee, WI.

Research in Behavioral
Parent Training in Social Work:
A Review

Richard A. Polster
Richard F. Dangel
Robert Rasp

SUMMARY. A literature search of 10 years (1975-1985) of 13 prominent social work journals yielded 83 articles for a review of research in behavioral parent training in social work. The review showed social workers deliver an impressive array of services to a broad variety of parents and their children. The review also revealed that the articles generally lacked operational descriptions of interventions, empirical rigor, and reliably demonstrated results. In light of these findings, summary conclusions are made and recommendations for future directions for research in behavioral parent training in social work are suggested.

Our task: To critically review the latest clinical research pertinent to "Behavioral Parent Training in Social Work." First, we developed working definitions of "social work," "parent training," and "behavioral." We defined social work by its journals: we reviewed all articles in the major social work journals from 1975 through 1985. Table I lists the journals we included in our review. We defined parent training loosely to include any article that reported an attempt to influence parent child relationships or interactions. We defined an intervention as behavioral if the article specifically mentioned instructing a parent (or other respon-

Correspondence may be addressed to Richard A. Polster, PhD, Graduate School of Social Work, University of Texas at Arlington, P.O. Box 19129, Arlington, Texas 76019-0129.

37

Table I

Social Work Journals Reviewed, 1975-1985

Child Welfare

Clinical Social Work Journal

Journal of Social Service Research

Journal of Social Welfare

Public Welfare

Smith College Studies in Social Work

Social Casework

Social Service Review

Social Work

Social Work and Research Abstracts

Social Work in Education

Social Work in Health Care

Social Work with Groups

sible member such as foster parent, grandparent, or guardian) in a procedure generally associated with "behavioral." Examples of behavioral procedures include: time-out, positive reinforcement, restriction of privileges, rewards, points, tokens, etc. This netted us a total of 82 articles. Twenty-six articles instructed parents to employ a behavioral procedure. The remaining 56 stated or implied a goal of some parent or child behavior change.

Our selection approach, granted, leaves room for error. Obviously, social work research appears in many journals in addition to those included in our review; procedures other than those we selected may be considered behavioral; and articles that should have been included may have been overlooked. We believe, nevertheless, the included articles do provide a sufficient sample to summarize the state-of-the art in behavioral parent training in social work and to provide both a commentary and suggestions for future directions.

This review is divided into three sections. The first section describes several parent training intervention components. These components include the subjects, settings, intervention methods, service duration, and treatment goals. The second section examines issues in evaluation, including: experimental designs, measurement systems, and results. In the third section we summarize our findings and suggest directions for future behavioral parent training research in social work.

PARENT TRAINING INTERVENTION COMPONENTS

Subjects

The 83 articles that fit our classification scheme addressed a broad range of subjects. We found that almost half of the articles made the age of the children a contingency for parents' participation in parent training. Of the articles specifying age, 85% involved parents whose children were under 13 years old.

Sixty-seven of the articles dealt with parents of children with nonorganic failure to thrive (Koepke & Thyer, 1985; Moore, 1982); psychotic children (Cozzarelli & Sillin, 1984); juvenile offenders (Douds, Engelsgjerd & Collingwood, 1977); children acting-out in school (Jayarante, 1978); and children labelled "disturbed" (Bauer & Heinke, 1976). Only 15 of the articles focused on at-large parent populations, where participation was not contingent on the child displaying dysfunctional behavior.

We found a broad variety of parents represented in the literature. Eighteen percent of the articles included parents who had abused or neglected their children. In over 50% of the articles, mothers were the sole recipients of service. Both mothers and fathers were equally represented in 34% of the articles. Nearly a quarter of the studies, however, failed to specify fathers' involvement. To our surprise, of the 82 articles we reviewed, only one (Hardy, Santa & Mahon-Herrera, 1981) addressed the specific needs of minority group parents.

Settings

We found that practitioners conducted parent training in virtually every setting where parents and children are found. The majority of articles described parent training on an outpatient basis through clinics, hospitals, and schools. Outpatient parent training was also offered through residential treatment centers (five articles) and day-care programs (seven articles). Fourteen articles described parent training efforts that were conducted in clients' homes. Examples of home-based parent training include programs for: adolescents experiencing school difficulties and having problems with their parents (Jayarante, 1978); families of neglected or developmentally delayed children (Arch, 1978), and abusive and neglectful parents (Miller, Fein, Howe, Gaudio & Bishop, 1984).

Intervention Methods

Of the 83 articles we reviewed, only 16 discussed parent training as the sole intervention. In the 67 other articles, parent training was implemented in conjunction with a variety of interventions. For the most part, authors referred to these other interventions as individual, group, or family therapy for parents and their children. Lillesand (1977), for example, explained that she integrated parent training with individual, marital, or group therapy for parents, while she also employed individual or group therapy with their children.

Table II presents a frequency distribution of the parent training methods practitioners used. Formal instruction, used in 79% of

Table II

Frequency Distribution of Parent Training Methods

Method	Total[a]	Method	Total[a]
Formal Instruction	66	Written Material	11
Group Process	42	Role Play	10
Modeling	27	Video Tapes	6
Informal Instruction During Family Therapy	19	Audio Tapes	2
Homework Assignments	12		

[a]Many practitioners used more than one technique, so the total adds to more than 100%.

the articles, was the most common parent training method. Formal instruction was defined as practitioners lecturing clients regarding parenting issues, or practitioners directing clients to perform specific parenting behavior. The content of formal instruction was quite varied across articles. The most common topics that practitioners addressed included: communication techniques (e.g., Hirsch, Gailey & Schmerl, 1976), problem solving skills (e.g., Katz, 1979), child development (e.g., Kreech, 1975), and behavioral principles (e.g., Penn, 1978).

Group process, defined as clients participating in group discussions on parenting topics, was represented in 51% of the articles. Many practitioners explained that group process was beneficial because it offered parents the opportunity to compare their ideas, experiences, and concerns. The most common topic parents discussed in their groups included: the information presented by the practitioner, problems and successes with their children, and applications and modifications of parenting methods they practiced with their own children (e.g., Bauer & Heinke, 1976; Ross & Schreiber, 1975).

Modeling was paired with formal parenting instruction in 27 articles. Modeling was defined as practitioners demonstrating techniques they described in one-to-one interactions and lectures (e.g., Koepke & Thyer, 1985; Kreech, 1975; Miller, Fein, Howe, Gaudio & Bishop, 1984; Penn, 1978).

Practitioners employed informal parent training instruction in 19 articles. Informal parent training included a wide variety of information, suggestions, and directions that practitioners typically included as part of what they discussed as, "family therapy" (e.g., Burroughs; 1985; Hagen, 1983; Lesoff, 1975).

Twelve authors discussed homework assignments as at least one part of their parent training efforts. Katz (1979), for example, asked parents to count the number of "strokes" they gave, received, and needed during each week.

We found that in 11 articles, practitioners used written materials to assist in their parent training. Penn (1978), for example, used his own manual, *Changing Children's Behavior*, to enhance his formal instruction. Oppenheimer (1978) used Patterson's (1976) *Living with Children* as the basis for teaching specific parenting skills. Several practitioners used Gordon's (1975) *Par-*

ent Effectiveness Training materials with their clients (e.g., McNeil & McBride, 1979).

The majority of intervention descriptions showed that practitioners relied primarily on some sort of verbal instruction. In 10 articles, however, clinicians not only gave information, but they also had parents put their new knowledge into action by role playing (e.g., Katz, 1979; Vassil, 1978).

Our review found few practitioners using media technology in their parent training. Six articles discussed practitioners' videotape use as one part of their intervention. Mastria, Mastria, and Harkins (1979), for example, videotaped interactions between parents and their children. Practitioners then replayed the tape for parents, discussing alternatives to negative interactions that appeared on the tape. Two articles discussed the use of audio tapes as part of parent training (e.g., Bauer & Heinke, 1976).

Service Duration

We attempted to analyze the duration of parents' involvement in parent training. This information, unfortunately, was absent from many of the articles. Twenty-three of them did not indicate any treatment length at all. Thirty articles specified that the intervention was "long term" (more than six months). Of the remaining 30 articles, 79% lasted between six and 12 weeks. We drew only one conclusion from our analysis: interventions that were primarily educational were generally shorter term than approaches that practitioners labelled as some sort of "therapy."

The many different service durations and the great variety of intervention components that practitioners have used suggest they have been creative and adaptable in their parent training. Whether pairing parent training with other intervention components, or involving parents in long or short term treatment, clinicians were consistently trying to adapt and improve old methods and to find new ways to help parents improve their relationships with their children. Some practitioners, however, made it difficult for us to determine their treatment purpose.

Treatment Goals

We were surprised that we found so many articles that did not specify treatment goals. Twenty-five articles, in fact, made no mention of goals whatsoever. While the remaining 57 articles indicated some form of goal, they were typically stated in broad or unmeasurable terms. Some examples of nonoperational goals included: "provide the family with a milieu that is health oriented rather than problem oriented," "help the child and family live together," and "guide the parents in facilitating adjustment for their children."

Of the 57 articles that indicated goals, only 27 made any mention of specific parent training goals. The two most common parent training goals were (1) to teach parents to help their children behave more appropriately, and (2) to change feelings or attitudes about being a parent. Banchy and Canter (1979) provided an excellent operational example of the first type of parent training goal. One of their three stated objectives was that parents teach their children 80% of the tasks presented by the "parent-educator." Other parent training goals we found included parents' learning: developmental information, problem solving, and communication skills. We were disappointed to find so few operationalized goals. We suspected that without specified and measurable goals, outcome evaluation would surely suffer.

EVALUATION

To identify and catalog the different ways authors evaluated the outcomes of their parent training, we defined evaluation as: any discussion of parent or child behavior change as a result of practitioners' efforts. We considered evaluation, therefore, to include practitioner assertions such as, "Mr. Jones was better able to respond to his son at the end of treatment." While, at the other end on a continuum of systematic rigor, we also considered evaluation to include well controlled experimental designs and comprehensive measurement systems. LeCroy, Koeplin-LeCroy, and Long (1982), for example, evaluated their parent training work by employing single-case experimental designs, as well as, by using pre- and posttests to evaluate individuals' behavior change and program effectiveness.

Experimental Designs

Of the 83 parent training articles we reviewed, only 11 specified some form of experimental design. Of these 11 articles, five described single subject experimental procedures. Of these five, three used multiple baseline designs (e.g., Polster & Pinkston, 1979). Two practitioners used (AB) designs, comparing frequencies of behavior during baseline to frequencies during intervention. The remaining six articles that discussed experimental designs used control or comparison groups and statistical analysis of the differences in pretest and posttest scores (e.g., Philipp & Siefert, 1979).

Measurement Systems

Although most clinicians did not specify experimental designs, many of them (38%) attempted to measure some behavior that may have been effected by parent training. Sixteen articles described practitioners' attempts to directly measure the effects of their parenting instructions, or recommendations, on parents' behavior. Pinkston and Herbert-Jackson (1975), for example, examined whether parents trained to use time-out, applied the skill correctly at appropriate times. Other authors tried to obtain a more general picture of the effects of their parent training. Wolf (1983), for example, collected parents' self-report data on their: using negative actions, adhering to logical and natural consequences, and children's obedience. In another attempt to evaluate the effects of parent training, Dooley, Prochaska, and Klibanoff (1983) and Pill (1981), for example, administered "satisfaction with service" questionnaires to parents at their final meeting.

Of the 32 authors who tried to measure some effect of their intervention, 11 used standardized measures. Some of these measures included the: Coopersmith Self-Esteem Inventory (Schofield, 1979), Iowa Test of Basic Skills (Polster & Pinkston, 1979), Caldwell Cooperative Preschool Inventory (Banchy &

Canter, 1979), Becker Adjective Checklist and Locke-Wallace Marital Inventory (Barth, Blythe, Schinke & Schilling, 1983).

Twenty authors attempted to measure change by nonstandardized means. Some of these practitioners employed nonstandard measures they developed specifically for their parent training work. Penn (1978), for example, administered his Child Behavior Inventory with parents to establish their pre- and post program impressions of their children's behavior. Neuhring, Abrams, Fike and Ostrowsky (1983) developed and standardized their own assessment instruments to evaluate their parenting interventions. Caseworkers completed an 11-item Parent-Child Interaction Checklist and a 10-item Health and Nutrition Activities Checklist based on their direct observations of each client family. The caseworkers completed these checklists at intake and at 90 day intervals thereafter.

RESULTS

Twenty-one percent (17) of the authors did not discuss results at all. Even though the majority of articles we reviewed did not demonstrate experimental control or systematically rigorous measurement, 35% of the authors asserted positive treatment effects based solely on their impressions. Some of these practitioners presented their assertions as conclusions to case studies. Most authors, however, presented no additional information, operationalized terms, or quantitative data to support claims of positive treatment effects such as, "improved ego strength," "reduced anxiety," "and increased self esteem."

Thirty six authors supported their claims of positive intervention effects through operational descriptions, and quantitative evidence. In nine articles, parents' quantitative or descriptive self reports on their, or their children's behavior, indicated improvement. Parents reported their children changed such behaviors as: tantrums, bedwetting, school performance, and playing with peers (Titkin & Cobb, 1983); violence (Mastria et al., 1979); and cooperation with parents (Wolf, 1983). Parents' self reports showed they improved their own parenting behaviors by: using social reinforcement and ignoring minor inappropriate child behaviors (LeCroy et al., 1982); eliminating assaults on their children (Mastria et al., 1979); and decreasing negative actions towards their children (Wolf, 1983).

Practitioners in 19 articles compared pre- to postintervention data to show positive results had occurred. Cautley (1980) reported clients improved many child rearing skills, including life maintenance, emotional nurturance, cognitive development, and socialization. In other examples, Moore (1982), found that of parents who had worked with her due to their infants' failure to thrive, none of the babies were rehospitalized for that problem. Koepke and Thyer (1985) also found positive results through their training of a parent of a nonorganic failure to thrive infant. Their subject's baby steadily gained and maintained weight after parent training. Banchy and Carter (1979), helped parents successfully teach their children school readiness tasks.

Results in the final nine articles were derived from well controlled studies that employed systematic measurement and data analysis. LeCroy and associates (1982), for example, found statistically significant changes in occurrence frequency of parental requests, siblings' fighting, chores completed, and whining. Burch and Mohr (1980) noted that participants in their Positive Parenting class changed their attitudes, perspectives, and knowledge about child care and development, while a control group did not make similar changes. In another study, Pinkston and Herbert-Jackson (1975) helped parents decrease their child's irrelevant and bizarre verbalizations. Finally, Barth and associates (1983) demonstrated that abusive parents who learned self-control procedures significantly increased their "positive self talk" and praise for managing hypothetical child problem situations. In this study, videotaped role plays of parent child interactions showed, among other things, parents' improved ability to keep calm during stressful situations and their decreased use of blaming statements.

We began our review with three strong biases regarding evaluation. First, practitioners should include evaluation as part of every intervention program. Second, evaluation is an inherent part of any research that employs behavioral procedures. Third, practitioners derive benefits from evaluation by sharing their results with other clinicians through professional publications. Furthermore, since the Council on Social Work Education

(CSWE) standards for graduate education require research coursework for all students, we thought our biases corresponded with a majority view in social work. Our review clearly demonstrated, however, that when it comes to journal publications, our evaluation biases represented a minority perspective. We found few articles that included quantitative evaluation, regardless of their application of behavioral parent training methods.

CONCLUSIONS

While our review represents only a small fraction of the diverse parenting services that are offered, social workers can be proud of the extent of services they make available to troubled parents and children. They provide parent training services in schools, mental health centers, social service agencies, hospitals, residential treatment centers, universities, and private clinics.

Many of the practitioners employ behavioral methods to teach parents ways to influence their children. Some of these behavioral techniques include: positive reinforcement contingent on appropriate behavior, time-out, differential reinforcement of other behavior, shaping, fading, and contracting.

Over the past 10 years, the social work parent training literature has begun to acknowledge that disruptions in parent-child relationships may be due to deficient parenting skills, not just a symptom of underlying parental psychological problems or marital discord. This recognition expands the treatment goals for social workers working with families in need. Scientifically proven laws of human behavior, once denied, often ignored by the profession, seem to be accepted and employed not only to train parents, but also as procedures for parents to use with their children. Social work can thank behaviorism for these major advances.

Regardless of the theoretical framework of the service provided, with few exceptions, the bulk of social work parent training articles provide little more than a sketchy description of the population served by the program, an even sketchier description of the service provided and the treatment aims, and far too often a dangerous and sweeping overstatement of results. Readers may erroneously conclude, "Hey, this worked!" without knowing what the "this" is or what "worked" means. Such a conclusion can stop any search for treatment methods that explain and demonstrate results. This state of affairs is unfortunate. It seems reasonable to assume that at least some of the interventions helped at least some of the time. We do not, however, find sufficient information in most of the articles that can help others replicate the interventions.

It is a great loss that so much service delivery occurs yet so little evidence of effectiveness accrues. Fortunately, human service research practitioners have begun to outline essential components to reverse this loss (Gambrill, 1983). First, social workers must begin to use measurement systems to evaluate parent training if they are to surpass the prevalent practice of offering only simple program descriptions. While a measurement system by itself is usually insufficient to allow for the making of causal statements (i.e., this parent training program caused these changes), it can tell the practitioner the magnitude of any change and whether the treatment failed. It also provides a comparison level, Without which any evaluation is impossible. Measurement systems do not require tremendous research expertise. Numerous textbooks describe various measurement tools (Mash & Terdal, 1981); some are devoted specifically to measuring changes in parent-child interactions (Forehand & McMahon, 1981). Computer software makes this task even easier (see, *Computers in Human Services* [journal]).

Second, clearer descriptions of the treatment and specification of treatment objectives will allow for replication by others. Replication permits the selection of programs that work and the disposal of others. As the field of parent training in social work stands right now, practitioners are left to frequently reinvent the wheel. Program descriptions and treatment objectives are typically so vague as to be useless. The importance of specificity in describing the treatment, as well as the treatment objectives, is well documented (Bloom & Fischer, 1982). Several texts are available to help the practitioner complete this step (Bloom & Fischer, 1982; Gambrill, 1983).

Finally, single subject experimental designs provide an important missing piece to the evaluation puzzle. No longer are huge numbers of randomly selected subjects required. Parent trainers can evaluate program effectiveness with their next client. Several excellent texts describe how to use single subject designs (Barlow, Hayes & Nelson, 1984; Barlow & Hersen, 1984). Numerous parent training articles provide models employing single subject designs in practice (see articles in the *Journal of Applied Behavior Analysis, Behavior Modification*, and the *Journal of Child Behavior Therapy*).

In a brilliant address presented at the *Conference on Practitioners as Evaluators of Direct Practice*, Gambrill (1985) identified numerous obstacles to incorporating evaluation methods into direct social work practice, and methods to attack these obstacles. Deficits in required skills and knowledge, inadequate support systems, and a lack of incentives constitute the primary obstacles to evaluation. Reducing fear, examining preferred explanations, encouraging clear thinking, providing required skills and knowledge, and arranging incentives will provide solutions to these obstacles.

Social work readers can facilitate the incorporation of evaluation into direct practice by displaying a healthy dose of skepticism (not cynicism) when reading articles. Asking questions like, "How does the author know that? What proof is offered? Couldn't that change be due to x, y, or z?" will encourage the systematic search for treatments that can be empirically demonstrated to work. Furthermore, authors may feel more inclined to attempt to provide answers to these very tough questions if they know readers demand them.

Journal editors must share this vital responsibility. They must set minimum standards for publication that include attempts at measurement and evaluation. They must also teach contributors to keep claims of program success within the boundaries of obtained data rather than determined by the practitioners' impressions. Articles should be categorized as program descriptions or program descriptions with evaluations; with publication priority being given to the latter. These recommended changes can help elevate the nature of social work publications to be more consistent with the much praised and desperately needed move towards social work as science.

REFERENCES

Arch, S. D. (1978). Older adults as home visitors modeling parenting for troubled families. *Child Welfare*, 57(9), 601-605.

Bauer, J. E. & Heinke, W. (1976). Treatment family care homes for disturbed foster children. *Child Welfare*, 55(7), 478-490.

Banchy, N. & Cantier, A. (1979). A home based parent education program. *Social Work in Education*, 1(2), 36-46.

Barth, R. P., Blythe, B. J., Schinke, S. P. & Schilling, R. F. (1983). Self-control training with maltreating parents. *Child Welfare*, 55(4), 313-324.

Barlow, D. A., Hayes, S. C. & Nelson, R. O. (1984). *The Scientist Practitioner*. New York: Pergamon.

Barlow, D. H. & Hersen, M. (1984). *Single Case Experimental Designs*, 2nd ed.; New York: Pergamon.

Bauer, J. E. & Heinke, W. (1976). *Child Welfare*, 55(7), 478-490.

Behavior Modification (Journal). Published by Sage.

Bloom, M. & Fischer, J. (1982). *Evaluating practice: Guidelines for the accountable professional*. Englewood Cliffs, NJ: Prentice Hall.

Burch, G. & Mohr, V. (1980). Evaluating a child abuse program. *Social Casework*, 61(2), 90-100.

Burroughs, C. H. (1985). Working with families of severely disturbed children in a day treatment setting. *Clinical Social Work Journal*, 13(2), 129-139.

Cautley, P. W. (1980). Treating dysfunctional families at home. *Social Work*, 25(5), 380-386.

Computers in Human Services (Journal). Published by Haworth Press. Richard Schoech, Editor.

Cozzarelli, L. A. & Silin, M. W. (1984). Therapeutic interventions with families with psychotic young children. *Clinical Social Work Journal*, 12(2), 140-151.

Dooley, B., Prochaska, J. M. & Klibanoff, P. (1983). "What next?": An educational program for parents of newborns. *Social Work in Health Care*, 8(4), 95-103.

Douds, A. F., Engelsgjerd, M. & Collingwood, T. R. (1977). Behavior contracting with youthful offenders and their parents. *Child Welfare*, 56(6), 409-417.

Forehand, R. & McMahon, R. (1981). *Helping the non-compliant child*. New York: Guilford.

Gambrill, E. (1983). *Casework: A competency-based approach*. Englewood-Cliffs, NJ: Prentice-Hall.

Gambrill, E. (1985). The state of the art in practice evaluation. Paper presented at the *Conference on Practitioners as Evaluators of Direct Practice*. University of Washington, Seattle. Washington, June 16, 17 & 18.

Gordon, T. (1985). *Parent effectiveness training: The tested new way to raise responsible children*. New York: Plume Books.

Hagen, J. V. (1983). One residential center's model for working with families. *Child Welfare*, 62(3), 233-241.

Hardy-Santa, C. & McMahon-Herrera, E. (1981). Adapting family therapy to the hispanic family. *Social Casework*, 62(3), 138-148.

Hirsch, J. S., Gailey, J. & Schmerl, E. (1976). A child welfare agency's program of service to children in their own homes. *Child Welfare*, 55(3), 193-204.

Jayarante, S. (1978). Behavioral intervention and family decision-making. *Social Work*, 23(1), 20-25.

Journal of Applied Behavior Analysis. Published by the Society for the Experimental Analysis of Behavior. Brian A. Iwata, Editor.

Journal of Child Behavior Therapy. Published by Haworth Press. Cyril Franks, Editor.

Katz, M. (1979). Communication workshop for parents. *Social Work in Education,* 2(1), 28-40.

Koepke, J. M. & Thyer, B. A. (1985). Behavioral treatment of failure-to-thrive in a two-year-old. *Child Welfare,* 64(5), 511-516.

Krecch, F. (1975). A residence for mothers and their babies. *Child Welfare,* 54(8), 581-592.

LeCroy, C. W., Koeplin-LeCroy, M. T. & Long, J. (1982). Preventive intervention through parent-training programs. *Social Work,* 4(2), 53-62.

Lesoff, R. (1975). Foster's technique: A systematic approach to family therapy. *Clinical Social Work Journal,* 3(1), 32-45.

Lillesand, D. B. (1977). A behavioral-psychodynamic approach to day treatment for emotionally disturbed children. *Child Welfare,* 56(9), 613-619.

Mash, E. J. & Terdal, L. G. (1981). *Behavioral assessment of childhood disorders.* New York: Guilford.

Mastria, E. O., Mastria, M. A. & Harkins, J. C. (1979). Treatment of child abuse by behavioral intervention: A case report. *Child Welfare,* 58(4), 253-261.

McNeil, J. S. & McBride, M. L. (1979). Group therapy with abusive parents. *Social Casework,* 60(1), 36-42.

Moore, J. B. (1982). Project thrive: A supportive treatment approach to the parents of children with nonorganic failure to thrive. *Child Welfare,* 61(6), 389-399.

Miller, K., Fein, E., Howe, G. W., Gaudio, C. & Bishop, G. V. (1984). Time-limited, goal-focused parent aide service. *Social Casework,* 65(8), 472-477.

Neuhring, E. M., Abrams, H. A., Fike, D. F. & Ostrowsky, E. F. (1983). Evaluating the impact of prevention programs aimed at children. *Social Work Research & Abstracts,* 19(2), 11-18.

Oppenheimer, A. (1978). Triumph over trauma in the treatment of child abuse. *Social Casework,* 59(6), 352-358.

Patterson, G. R. (1976). *Living with children: New methods for parents and teachers.* Champaign, IL: Research Press.

Penn, J. V. (1978). A model for training foster parents in behavior modification techniques. *Child Welfare,* 57(3), 175-180.

Philipp, C. & Siefert, K. (1979). A study of material participation in preschool programs for handicapped children and their families. *Social Work in Health Care,* 5(2), 165-175.

Pill, C. J. (1981). A family life education group for working with stepparents. *Social Casework,* 62(3), 159-166.

Pinkston, E. M. & Herbert-Jackson, E. W. (1975). Modification of irrelevant and bizarre verbal behavior using parents as therapists. *Social Service Review,* 49(1), 46-63.

Polster, R. A. & Pinkston, E. M. (1979). A delivery system for the treatment of underachievement. *Social Service Review,* 53(1), 35-55.

Ross, A. L. & Schreiber, L. J. (1975). Bellefaire's day treatment program: An interdisciplinary approach to the emotionally disturbed child. *Child Welfare,* 54(3), 183-194.

Schofield, R. (1979). Parent group education and student self-esteem. *Social Work in Education,* 1(2), 26-32.

Titkin, E. A. & Cobb, C. (1983). Treating post-divorce adjustment in latency age children: A focused group paradigm. *Social Work with Groups,* 6(2), 53-66.

Vassil, T. V. (1978). Residential family camping: Altering family patterns. *Social Casework,* 59(10), 605-613.

Wolf, M. C. M. (1983). Integrated family systems model for parent education. *Social Work in Education,* 5(3), 188-199.

Behavioral Social Work
with Obsessive-Compulsive Disorder

Gail Steketee

SUMMARY. The symptomatology of obsessive-compulsive disorder is described and its negative impact on daily functioning is noted. The outcome of the application of various forms of behavioral treatment, including systematic desensitization, imaginal exposure, aversion treatment and thought-stopping is discussed with reference to theoretical formulations of the function of obsessions and compulsions vis-à-vis anxiety. Behavioral treatment via a combination of exposure to feared situations and response prevention or blocking of ritualistic behavior has proven to be the treatment of choice for this disorder. It is described here in some detail and suggestions regarding clinical issues in conducting this treatment are given. Factors identified as possible predictors of outcome include depression, anxious mood state, patients' beliefs in the probability of feared consequences, social functioning, motivation level and therapist characteristics. It is concluded that exposure and response prevention has substantially improved the prognosis of clients with obsessive-compulsive disorder but that programs aimed at maintenance of gains over time are needed.

In the past decade, behavioral forms of psychotherapeutic treatment have drawn increasing attention from social workers who are engaged in the direct treatment of individuals with psychosocial problems. Social workers have achieved favorable outcomes using behavioral methods with severely anxiety disordered patients, including simple phobics (e.g., Sank, 1976;

Preparation of this manuscript was supported by NIMH Grant No. 31634, awarded to Edna B. Foa, PhD, Temple University, Department of Psychiatry.

Reprint requests should be addressed to the author at Boston University, School of Social Work, 264 Bay State Road, Boston, MA 02215.

53

Thyer, 1981), social phobics (e.g., Hudson, 1974), agoraphobics (e.g., Hudson, 1974) and obsessive-compulsives (Steiner, Welber, Arder & Carrol, 1980; Steketee, Foa & Grayson, 1982). For a review of this literature see Thyer (1983). The present paper summarizes the research findings with respect to behavioral treatment of the last group, obsessive-compulsives. Following a description of this disorder, a theoretical framework for conceptualizing and treating obsessions and compulsions is presented. Outcome data on several behavioral treatment methods is presented and the most successful of these interventions, exposure and response prevention, is described in some detail. Variables which are predictive of success and failure with this treatment method are discussed with particular reference to the patient's social context and its impact on long-term outcome.

DESCRIPTION OF
OBSESSIVE-COMPULSIVE DISORDER

According to the DSM-III (1980), individuals with an obsessive-compulsive disorder are afflicted with persistent intrusive and disturbing obsessive thoughts, images or impulses which are ego dystonic. These symptoms are typically accompanied by extensive avoidance behaviors and compulsive actions performed to relieve the discomfort provoked by the obsessions. Two forms of compulsive behavior predominate: washing and/or cleaning rituals and checking rituals. The obsessive concerns of washers and cleaners typically center around fears of "contamination" from such diverse sources as bathroom germs, food crumbs, household chemicals, cancer patients or even one's hometown. Individuals with checking rituals commonly fear making important mistakes (such as leaving the stove on, failing to lock doors or windows, throwing out important papers) or harming others (e.g., unintentionally running over someone in a car, feeding the family moldy food without realizing it). Less common forms of compulsions include repetitious actions such as retracing one's steps or dressing and undressing repeatedly and ordering rituals usually performed to achieve a satisfying sense of symmetry of objects. Covert or cognitive compulsions may involve repeated praying, counting or thinking "good" thoughts to offset "bad" ones.

Compulsive behaviors often consume many hours a day. As they become increasingly elaborate, individuals with this disorder develop extensive methods to avoid their feared situations and thereby avert the need to ritualize. Often the anticipated harm associated with obsessional fears constitutes the primary cause for the patient's discomfort. Most individuals with washing rituals worry that contamination will result in disease, physical debilitation or death to themselves or others. Those with checking or repeating compulsions fear being responsible for physical harm (e.g., leaving the stove on and thereby burning the house down, losing control and stabbing one's daughter) or psychological harm (e.g., setting the table incorrectly and being criticized by a significant other, writing "I am a homosexual" on a check and losing others' respect).

It should be noted that obsessive-compulsive disorder is distinguished here from compulsive personality style. The latter is characterized by orderliness, rigidity, indecisiveness and perfectionism; parsimony and punctuality are included in some definitions. Although such traits are present in a proportion of individuals with an obsessive-compulsive disorder, they are by no means a defining characteristic. Indeed, Rosenberg (1967) found that only 25 percent of his sample exhibited such personality traits. Although an association between obsessional symptoms and traits has been claimed, its nature and extent remains unclear (Pollack, 1979; Slade, 1974).

Obsessional thoughts and compulsive behaviors are found in very mild form in as many as 80 percent of "normal" individuals (Rachman & DeSilva, 1978; Salkovskis & Harrison, 1984). In its severe form, however, obsessional thinking accompanied by extensive ritualistic behaviors and avoidance patterns often interferes with satisfactory functioning across many personal and interpersonal spheres.

As Rachman and Hodgson (1980) point out:

> the presence in the family of a severely obsessional person can distort the lives of all of its members. As the incapacitation of the affected member spreads, the demands made on spouse, parents and children increase. Not only are they required to take over many of the patient's functions—do-

mestic, personal, financial and social—they also have to devote increasing time and effort to the protection and comforting of the affected person. In cases of severe and chronic disorders, the social, personal and financial damage to the entire family can be extensive and irreversible. (p. 62)

In a sample of 72 adult obsessive-compulsives (55 percent female) who sought treatment from the Temple University Department of Psychiatry since 1975, about two-thirds were unable to complete their education, work in paid employment or carry out household duties satisfactorily. Only half were married. Males predominated in the single group, with more than two-thirds living with their parents or relatives, despite the relatively high mean age for the sample of 34 years (s.d. = 10.6 years). Many were severely restricted in their social activities, depending heavily on family members for emotional and structural support and in many cases for help with their rituals. Yet the intelligence level of this group is above the norm; more than 60 percent had some college training or graduate education. Such figures are typical of obsessive-compulsives studied in other centers (Kringlen, 1970; Ingram, 1961).

THEORETICAL CONCEPTUALIZATION OF OBSESSIVE-COMPULSIVE DISORDER

Although it is customary to refer to thoughts and images as "obsessions" and to repetitious actions as "compulsions," this classification according to the modality (cognition vs. overt behavior) rather than the function of the symptoms is not useful and can be misleading (Foa & Steketee, 1979). Rather, a distinction which rests on the relationship between anxiety or discomfort and symptomatology has considerable relevance for treatment as will be demonstrated shortly. Accordingly, obsessions are viewed as cognitions or actions which increase discomfort and compulsions are defined as overt behaviors or cognitions which are carried out to reduce the discomfort provoked by the obsessions. Although the acquisition of obsessive-compulsive symptoms is not well understood, the process by which they are maintained is better documented. It is generally accepted that the reduction of anxiety brought about by rituals serves to negatively reinforce such behaviors and thereby to increase the likelihood that they will be performed in the future (Foa, Steketee & Ozarow, 1985). The degree to which cognitive factors may be involved in acquisition and maintenance is still largely unknown (for review see Foa & Kozak, 1985; Steketee & Foa, 1985).

REVIEW OF TREATMENTS

Obsessive-compulsive disorders have long been considered among the most intractable of the neurotic disorders. Breitner (1960) noted that "most of us are agreed that the treatment of obsessional states is one of the most difficult tasks confronting the psychiatrist and many of us consider it hopeless" (p. 32). Traditional psychotherapy has had limited success in ameliorating obsessive-compulsive symptomatology (Black, 1974). In a sample of 90 inpatients, Kringlen (1965) found that only 20 percent had improved at a 13 to 20-year follow-up. More favorable but still unsatisfactory results were reported by Grimshaw (1965): 40 percent of an outpatient sample were improved one to 14 years after treatment.

EARLY FORMS OF BEHAVIORAL TREATMENTS

Some improvement in the prognostic picture emerged with the application of treatments derived from learning theories. Two types of methods have been employed: (1) exposure procedures aimed at reducing anxiety or discomfort and (2) blocking or punishing techniques directed at decreasing the frequency of either obsessive thoughts or ritualistic behaviors. (For a detailed review, see Foa, Steketee & Ozarow, 1985.)

The most commonly employed form of exposure treatment was systematic desensitization in which patients were briefly and gradually exposed to feared situations while practicing relaxation procedures. Although this procedure has been highly effective for simple phobics (e.g., Cooper, Gelder & Marks, 1965; Gelder, Marks & Wolfe, 1967), for obsessive-compulsives it produced improvement in only 30 to 40 percent of cases (Beech

& Vaughn, 1978; Cooper, Gelder & Marks, 1965). Several other treatment procedures utilizing prolonged exposure to feared cues (e.g., paradoxical intention, imaginal flooding, satiation and aversion relief) have also been employed with this population. Examined largely through case reports, these procedures have produced improvement rates of 60 percent or less, with the exception of aversion relief which proved effective to varying degrees for each of five patients.

The second set of treatment methods, blocking or punishing procedures, includes thought-stopping and various forms of aversion therapy. Thought-stopping has proven largely ineffective for obsessive-compulsive symptoms, with only one-third of cases improved in controlled studies. Aversion therapy via electrical shock, the snapping of a rubber band on the wrist or covert sensitization has yielded somewhat better results. However, findings are based on case reports and outcome studies conducted on very small sample sizes and must be considered only suggestive.

In the research discussed above, investigators rarely attempted to match the treatment procedure to the target symptom or to direct treatment at both obsessions and compulsions. If, as suggested previously, obsessions evoke anxiety and compulsions reduce it, it follows that treatments should be directed simultaneously at decreasing obsessive anxiety and suppressing compulsive behaviors. With the development of exposure and response prevention procedures these shortcomings were addressed. This program has proven highly effective and has become the treatment of choice for this disorder. A summary of the research on this procedure follows.

Exposure and Response Prevention

Meyer, Levy and Schnuner (1974) reported on a therapeutic program consisting of two basic components: (1) Direct *exposure* to objects or situations which provoke obsessional fears and (2) *response prevention* or preventing the compulsive behaviors. The results were remarkable: of the 15 patients treated with this program, 10 were rated as much improved or symptom-free and five were improved. Only two patients relapsed during the follow-up period. With these findings, interest in other methods of treatment was largely eclipsed and variants of *in vivo* exposure and response prevention have been investigated in some 20 studies to date. The overall success rates for this combination of behavioral procedures have been consistently high—about 75 percent of patients improved markedly with these treatments (for reviews see Emmelkamp, 1982; Foa, Steketee & Ozarow, 1985; Rachman & Hodgson, 1980). The addition of imaginal exposure to *in vivo* exposure produced similar if not somewhat better results (Foa & Goldstein, 1978; Steketee, Foa & Grayson, 1982).

At present, then, exposure *in vivo* and response prevention, sometimes with the addition of imaginal exposure, have been adopted as the treatment of choice for obsessive-compulsive ritualizers. Is it necessary, however, to apply all three procedures? Studies examining the role of each component are described below.

Differential Effects of Exposure and Response Prevention

The effectiveness of prolonged exposure procedures in reducing phobic fears is well established (Foa & Chambless, 1978; Grayson, Foa & Steketee, 1982; Nunes & Marks, 1975). If rituals are needed only because they reduce obsessional anxiety, then perhaps prolonged exposure alone would relieve both obsessions and compulsions, and response prevention would be unnecessary. Contrary to this hypothesis, Mills, Agras, Barlow and Mills (1973), studying five single cases, found that exposure alone produced either no change or an increase in compulsions and urges to ritualize, whereas response prevention alone virtually eliminated ritualistic behavior. Similar results were obtained in other single case experiments (Turner, Hersen, Bellack & Wells, 1979; Turner, Hersen, Bellack, Andrasik & Capparell, 1980) and in group studies (Foa, Steketee & Milby, 1980; Foa, Steketee, Grayson, Turner & Latimer, 1984). Deliberate exposure decreased anxiety to feared "contaminants" more than did merely blocking the compulsive washing. Conversely, ritualistic behavior was reduced more by response prevention than by exposure. Patients who received both procedures benefitted most on measures of both obsessional anxiety and time spent washing. corresponding changes were observed in general functioning.

Is imaginal exposure (flooding) effective in reducing obsessional symptoms and does it add to the utility of direct exposure *in vivo*? The literature suggests that for relief of specific phobias, actual confrontation with feared situations is superior to exposure in fantasy. It is reasonable to expect, then, that when obsessive fear is evoked primarily by concrete phobic objects such as urine or chemicals, exposure *in vivo* will produce greater gains than imaginal exposure. But for many obsessive-compulsives, anxiety is produced by both tangible cues from the environment and by anticipation of the harmful consequences (such as disease or the house burning down) that might follow. Exposure to these latter concerns can be accomplished only in fantasy. Consider the patient who constantly checks his rear view mirror and retraces his auto route because he is afraid he has inadvertently run over someone. Requiring him to drive without checking exposes him to the concrete road cues but may not provoke the portion of his fears that center around being responsible for actually hitting a pedestrian and leaving him behind to die. If it is important to match the content of the therapeutic exposure situation to a patient's internal fear model (as suggested by Lang, 1979), then those who fear harmful consequences which cannot be produced in reality should improve more with the addition of imaginal exposure.

To study this issue, patients who received exposure *in vivo* were compared with those who were given both exposure *in vivo* and in fantasy for the same time period (Foa, Steketee, Turner & Fisher, 1980; Steketee, Foa & Grayson, 1982). Both groups received response prevention. The two groups did not differ immediately after the intensive treatment but the addition of imaginal exposure did significantly improve the maintenance of such gains. Forty percent of those who received exposure *in vivo* only relapsed, whereas only 19 percent of the combined group lost gains (Steketee, Foa & Grayson, 1982). It appears, then, that when feared disasters are not directly addressed, the reduction of discomfort to environmental situations may be only temporary, perhaps because the core of the fear, i.e., concern with future catastrophes, has not changed.

In summary, the results of the studies discussed above argue for the use of deliberate *in vivo* exposure in combination with response prevention in the treatment of obsessive-compulsives. They also suggest that imaginal exposure be added for those who manifest fears of future catastrophes.

CLINICAL IMPLEMENTATION OF EXPOSURE AND RESPONSE PREVENTION

The treatment program for obsessive-compulsive disorders consists of three stages: an information gathering period, an intensive exposure/response prevention phase and a follow-up maintenance period. These are summarized below and detailed extensively in Steketee and Foa (1985).

Information Gathering Period

The goals of the first interviews with the patient are to establish a diagnosis and to collect information pertinent to treatment planning. To do so, the therapist solicits highly specific information about concrete situations which provoke anxiety in order to identify the basic sources of concern and possible harm associated with them. For example, a patient feared and avoided grass, dogs, shoes and garden tools because all were associated with contact with dog feces, the source of the obsessive anxiety. Contact with dog feces was thought to pose a risk of worms or other diseases to the patient's child.

Knowledge of both passive avoidance and active escape behaviors, that is, rituals, is essential in order to prohibit them during treatment, since even minor avoidances may serve to maintain obsessive fear. Examples of more subtle avoidance patterns include sidestepping brown spots on the sidewalk which may be possible dog feces and wearing slip-on shoes to avoid having to touch laces or buckles. Common forms of ritualistic behavior have already been described. Less obvious ones include wiping with alcohol or spraying with lysol, repeatedly requesting reassurance, and cognitive rituals, such as praying, thinking "good" thoughts or listing events mentally. The relationship among rituals, the sources of fear and passive avoidance should be ascertained. On the basis of the above information a treatment program can be designed.

Exposure. As noted earlier, actual exposure is recommended over imaginal techniques for external fears. Although the speed with which the most disturbing situation is confronted matters little (Boersma, Dem Hengst, Dekkar & Emmelkamp, 1976), most patients prefer gradual exposure. Usually, then, a five or six step hierarchy is employed, commencing exposure treatment with a moderately fearful object or situation and progressing to highly disturbing ones. Modelling by the therapist of contact with feared situations was not found to enhance the effectiveness of exposure, although some patients found it helpful (Rachman, Marks & Hodgson, 1973). For these individuals, then, the therapist demonstrates how to touch or hold the feared items. Longer periods of exposure have been found superior to brief interrupted ones (Rabavilas, Boulougouris & Stefanis, 1976). But unfortunately, little information about the optimal exposure time is available, nor do we know the best point at which to terminate an exposure session. For obsessive-compulsives, one to two hour sessions of continuous exposure have proven sufficient to permit anxiety reduction (Grayson, Foa & Steketee, 1982). Discussion of unrelated issues or distraction activities should be avoided since distraction of attention was associated with less anxiety reduction across sessions (Grayson, Foa & Steketee, 1982).

Imaginal exposure or "flooding" is employed to reduce fears of anticipated future disasters. Scenes of an hour or more duration are presented by the therapist according to a predesigned hierarchy of distress level. Included in these images are concrete cues (e.g., walking into a public bathroom), the patient's response (e.g., feeling shakey or heart racing) and feared consequences (e.g., becoming ill and receiving a diagnosis of leukemia). Presentations of such images are repeated for several sessions until discomfort declines.

Response prevention. The application of deliberate exposure interferes with obsessive-compulsives' ability to passively avoid their feared object: one cannot both avoid and confront one's fears at the same time. But exposure does not eliminate compulsions, and therefore response prevention must be implemented. The strictness of response prevention has varied across studies. In the treatment program at Temple University, washers are requested to refrain from all washing and cleaning except for one ten-minute shower every three to five days. Checkers are permitted a single check of only those items which are normally checked after use, such as stoves and door locks. Patients in other programs (e.g., Rachman, Hodgson & Marks, 1971) are permitted to wash normally but encouraged to avoid such washing for several hours following exposure. Both programs have been similarly effective, but no direct comparison of these methods has been conducted and thus the optimal degree of restriction is not known. The amount of supervision of the patient during treatment (whether 24-hour monitoring or none at all) also seems to affect outcome minimally, but again no direct comparison has been undertaken. In the Temple University program, patients are requested to designate a supervisor at home whose task is to provide support and encouragement to resist urges to ritualize. Physical force is never employed to prevent ritualistic behavior.

Cognitive rituals are more difficult to prevent, possibly because they are less identifiable than overt rituals and therefore less under the patient's control. Blocking techniques such as thought-stopping, aversion treatment and distraction may be of help, but as yet, information regarding the efficacy of these methods for covert symptoms is not available. In using such blocking procedures with cognitive rituals, it is important to distinguish between obsessions which increase anxiety and cognitive compulsions which reduce it, since the former require exposure to allow for anxiety reduction.

Treatment issues. Intensive treatment for a short period of time followed by weekly sessions as needed appears to be a highly effective therapy program for obsessive-compulsives (Steketee, Foa & Kozak, 1985). Daily sessions employed in some outcome studies (e.g., Foa et al., 1984; Marks, Stern, Mawson, Cobb & McDonald, 1980) may not be feasible in routine clinical practice. Clinical experience suggests that once-weekly sessions are probably not adequate for most patients, but two to three sessions per week may produce satisfactory results. Assistance from trainees or paraprofessionals may be enlisted to aid in exposure *in vivo* treatment. At times we have successfully conducted treatment using two therapists who alternated exposure sessions with two patients who had similar symptoms. Patients were seen jointly, thereby economizing on the therapist's time.

When confronted with a description of the exposure/response prevention treatment program, about 25 percent of obsessive-compulsives decline to participate (Foa, Steketee, Grayson & Doppelt, 1983). Only a few of those who elect to enter treatment fail to abide by the agreed-upon rules. In such cases the patient is encouraged to stop treatment and to return whenever he or she feels prepared to follow the instructions. Permitting patients to continue in an inadequate treatment is a substantial disservice, since it is likely to lead to failure (Foa, Grayson, Steketee, Turner & Latimer, 1983) and to loss of hope about future prospects for improvement.

Hospitalization is rarely required for exposure/response prevention treatment but may be indicated if patients live too far to commute to sessions or if the home environment is deemed unsupportive of efforts to improve. Hospitalization may be contraindicated when rituals are performed *only* in an environment for which the patient feels responsible. Those who repeatedly check to protect their family from burglary or fire rarely concern themselves with such responsibilities in the hospital where it is deemed the staff's duty to protect the environment. In such cases treatment should be conducted while the patient remains in his/her home setting.

As Steketee and Foa (1985) suggest, early in the data-gathering phase, the therapist is advised to initiate at least one session in which important family members (typically the spouse/partner or parents) attend. Family members' attitudes and interactions with the patient can be assessed with respect to their potential impact on the immediate and long term therapeutic process. The therapist can educate members about the disorder and its treatment and suggest methods for dealing with the patient's symptoms. Depending on the symptomatology, some patients may require assistance from their spouse, parents, friends or even clergy or family doctor. Such aid is particularly valuable when the patient's incessant requests for reassurance of these individuals constitute a compulsion and thus require refusal in order to effectively block this maladaptive strategy for reducing anxiety.

Similarly, for hospitalized patients regular consultation with nursing staff involved in assisting with the treatment regimen is needed. Placing a patient on a ward in which staff are not sympathetic to his or her struggles with anxiety or to the importance of following the treatment plan will obviously be detrimental to outcome.

COGNITIVE TREATMENT
OF OBSESSIVE-COMPULSIVE DISORDER

Although there is evidence for cognitive impairments in obsessive-compulsives (Steketee & Foa, 1985), efforts to treat these individuals with cognitive methods have not fared well. A few case studies have obtained positive outcomes using cognitive restructuring (e.g., Robertson, Wendiggenson & Kaplan, 1983; Salkovskis & Warwick, 1985), but the only reported controlled group study failed to find an effect of self-instructional training on obsessive-compulsive symptoms (Emmelkamp, Van der Helm, van Zanten & Plochg, 1980). The lack of impact of cognitive treatments may be due to their failure to address those aspects of cognitive impairment which are specific to obsessive-compulsive disorders. Such impairments may include exaggerated estimates of the probability of harm and misclassification or categorization of situations (Steketee & Foa, 1985).

PREDICTORS OF OUTCOME

Although the majority of obsessive-compulsives show considerable gains following exposure and response prevention, some 25 to 30 percent are unsuccessful in reducing their target symptoms. What characteristics distinguish those who succeed from those who fail? As noted earlier, incomplete exposure and response prevention whether instigated by the therapist or by the patient (through failure to comply), is likely to result in failure or relapse (Foa et al., 1983b).

Several authors have noted that the presence of severe depression hampers the effectiveness of exposure treatment (e.g., Boulougouris, 1977; Foa, Grayson & Steketee, 1982). Studies using tricyclic antidepressants for obsessive-compulsives have provided some support for this notion (e.g., Marks et al., 1980). However, recent findings from a prospective study conducted in our laboratory indicate that the tricyclic drug imipramine reduced depression without a corresponding decline in obsessions or compulsions (Foa, Steketee, Kozak & Dugger, 1985). Further, the level of depression did not predict outcome at post-treatment or at follow-up (Steketee, Foa & Kozak, 1985). These findings, as well as those of other investigators (e.g., Mavissakalian, Turner, Michelson & Jacob, 1985; Mawson, Marks & Ramm, 1982), suggest that the relationship between depression and obsessive-compulsive symptoms is more complex than initially thought and that high levels of depression in obsessive-compulsive patients are not necessarily predictive of failure.

Similarly, high levels of *general* anxiety or tension were not found to result consistently in failure (Foa et al., 1983b; Mawson, Marks & Ramm, 1982) although low initial anxiety was associated with a successful outcome (Foa et al., 1983b). The patient's anxiety response *during* exposure sessions has been linked to outcome in the following manner: those who reported high anxiety when first presented with their most feared obsessional situation tended to show more anxiety reduction during exposure sessions as well as across sessions (Foa et al., 1984) and to improve more after treatment.

A further stumbling block in treatment may be the patient's *belief system* regarding the likelihood that their feared consequence will in fact materialize. Whereas most patients are aware of the senselessness of their fears, a rare few will assert that the disaster they expect is highly probable unless they protect themselves by ritualizing. Foa (1979) observed that such individuals did not habituate to feared contaminants, either within an exposure session or across sessions. Unfortunately, reliable or valid measures of the degree of conviction in obsessive fears have not yet been developed and thus the validity of these observations has not been adequately tested.

Aspects of the individual's social functioning appear to bear on outcome, particularly at follow-up. Poor social functioning (e.g., lack of friendships or socializing outside of the family) prior to treatment was associated with *greater* change six months after treatment (Steketee, Foa & Kozak, 1985). This surprising association seems to be explained by the finding that *improvement* in social functioning during treatment was related to better long term gains. Certainly, those who function poorly at the outset have more opportunity to improve than those who are already functioning well.

Obsessive-compulsives with more cohesive marital relationships fared better after treatment (Hafner, 1982; Schwartz, 1982). Similarly, improvement in the quality of interaction with family members at post-treatment was found related to better long term outcome (Steketee, Foa & Kozak, 1985). Although clinicians have suggested that family members' reactions to patients' symptoms during and after treatment are important in recovery, no data on this issue is yet available. As Steketee and Foa (1985) have noted, family members have typically experienced intense frustration at the patient's irrational behavior and many are impatient, expecting treatment to result in rapid and complete symptom remission. Conversely, some may continue to "protect" the patient from formerly upsetting situations, thus reinforcing avoidance behaviors. Years of accommodation to the patient's peculiar requests have established patterns which are difficult to break and may foster relapse. Interventions directed at these difficulties may be required in such cases.

Being employed and satisfied with work was associated with better outcome (Schwartz, 1982). Many obsessive-compulsives have become occupationally nonfunctional as their symptoms usurped an increasing proportion of their lives. Since successful treatment leaves them with a considerable void in their daily routine, assistance in acquiring new skills and in planning both social and occupational activities may be needed to prevent relapse.

Consistent with findings reported for other anxiety disorders, both Foa et al. (1983b) and Rachman (1983) have commented anecdotally on the importance of a commitment to treatment in enhancing success. Steketee, Foa and Kozak (1985) observed that although a questionnaire measure of motivation for change was not correlated with outcome, attributing change after treatment to one's own willpower (versus medication, therapist, other support) was positively related to outcome three months later. Methods for increasing motivation and self-attribution have not been studied; it is likely that they are influenced by complex interactions among such factors as social environment, mood-state and beliefs and attitudes.

Characteristics of the therapist have also been implicated as prognostic factors. Therapist qualities of warmth, positive regard and empathy have long been recognized as important in psychotherapeutic treatment (e.g., Traux & Carkuff, 1967). With respect to exposure and response prevention, a study by Rabavilas, Boulougouris and Perissaki (1979) found that obsessive-compulsives who rated their therapists as respectful, understanding, interested, encouraging, challenging and explicit improved more; therapist's permissiveness, tolerance and gratification of dependency needs were associated with a negative outcome. Informal observations have led Marks, Hodgson and Rachman (1975) to suggest that "this treatment requires a good *patient-therapist working relationship*, and a sense of humor helps patients over difficult situations" (p. 360). Although it has been demonstrated that continuous therapist involvement during exposure treatment is not essential for a positive outcome (Emmelkamp & Kraanen, 1977), the therapist's presence may be needed to initiate difficult exposures and to encourage and challenge patients to continue in the face of considerable discomfort.

CONCLUDING COMMENTS

The application of behavioral treatment via exposure and response prevention has profoundly improved the prognostic picture for obsessive-compulsives. Two-thirds to three-quarters of patients have benefitted considerably from this treatment program over the long term. Unfortunately, however, patients rarely find themselves entirely symptom-free at the completion of this regimen and improvement does not endure for about 25 percent of patients (Foa et al., 1983a). For these individuals and their families, failure and relapse is costly in money, effort and hope. Relapse is most common among those patients who are only partially improved at the end of treatment, and for those whose impaired social and employment situation does not change. Adverse mood states such as depression and anxiety may also bear on outcome. As Wodarski and Bagarozzi (1979) suggest,

> the role of social workers in the process of ensuring maintenance of gains will be substantial [since] we are the professionals who are in the best position to affect the individual's environment . . . to ensure that sufficient reinforcements are provided and to help the individual practice the requisite behavior in the desired contexts. (p. 318)

With our present state of knowledge it is perhaps most important that we develop programs for maintenance of gains following exposure treatment. Such programs should focus on the patient's interpersonal and occupational adjustment and on providing support in their struggle to progress from a non-functional to a healthy lifestyle.

REFERENCES

American Psychiatric Association (1980). *Diagnostic and statistical manual of mental disorders*, 3rd ed.; Washington, DC: Author.

Beech, H. R. & Vaughn, M. (1978). *Behavioural treatment of obsessional states*. New York: Wiley.

Black, A. (1974). The natural history of obsessional neurosis. In H. R. Beech (Ed.), *Obsessional states*, pp. 19-54. London: Methuen.

Boersma, K., Den Hengst, S., Dekker, J. & Emmelkamp, P. M. G. (1976). Exposure and response prevention: A comparison with obsessive-compulsive patients. *Behaviour Research and Therapy, 14*, 19-24.

Boulougouris, J. C. (1977). Variables affecting the behaviour of obsessive-compulsive patients treated by flooding. In J. C. Boulougouris & A. Rabavilas (Eds.), *Studies in phobic and obsessive-compulsive disorders*, pp. 73-84. Oxford: Pergamon Press.

Breitner, C. (1960). Drug therapy in obsessional states and other psychiatric problems. *Diseases of the Nervous System, 21*, 31-35.

Cooper, J. E., Gelder, M. G. & Marks, I. M. (1965). The results of behavior therapy in 77 psychiatric patients. *British Medical Journal, 1*, 1222-1225.

Emmelkamp, P. M. G. (1982). *Phobic and obsessive-compulsive disorders. Theory, Research and Practice*. New York: Plenum Press.

Emmelkamp, P. M. G. & Kraaner, J. (1977). Therapist-controlled exposure *in vivo* versus self-controlled exposure *in vivo*: A comparison with obsessive-compulsive patients. *Behaviour Research and Therapy, 15*, 491-495.

Emmelkamp, P. M. G., van der Helm, M., van Zanten, B. L. & Plochg, I. (1980). Contributions of self-instructional training to the effectiveness of exposure *in vivo*: A comparison with obsessive-compulsive patients. *Behaviour Research and Therapy, 18*, 61-66.

Foa, E. B. (1979). Failure in treating obsessive-compulsives. *Behaviour Research and Therapy, 17*, 169-176.

Foa, E. B. & Chambless, D. L. (1978). Habituation of subjective anxiety during flooding in imagery. *Behaviour Research and Therapy*, *16*, 391-399.

Foa, E. B. & Goldstein, A. (1978). Continuous exposure and complete response prevention of obsessive-compulsive neurosis. *Behaviour Therapy*, *9*, 821-829.

Foa, E. B., Grayson, J. B. & Steketee, G. (1982). Depression, habituation and treatment outcome in obsessive-compulsives. In J. C. Boulougouris (Ed.), *Practical applications of learning theories in psychiatry*. New York: Wiley.

Foa, E. B., Grayson, J. B., Steketee, G. S., Doppelt, H. G., Turner, R. M. & Latimer, P. R. (1983a). Success and failure in the behavioral treatment of obsessive-compulsives. *Journal of Consulting and Clinical Psychology*, *51*, 287-297.

Foa, E. B. & Kozak, M. J. (1985). Treatment of anxiety disorders: Implications for psychopathology. In A. H. Tuma & J. D. Maser (Eds.), *Anxiety and the anxiety disorders*. Hillsdale, NY: Lawrence Erlbaum Associates.

Foa, E. B., Steketee, G., Grayson, J. B. & Doppelt, H. G. (1983b). Treatment of obsessive-compulsives: When do we fail? In E. B. Foa & P. M. G. Emmelkamp (Eds.), *Failures in behavior therapy*. New York: Wiley.

Foa, E. B., Steketee, G., Grayson, J. B., Turner, R. M. & Latimer, P. R. (1984). Deliberate exposure and blocking of obsessive-compulsive rituals: Immediate and long-term effects. *Behavior Therapy*, *15*, 450-472.

Foa, E. B., Steketee, G., Kozak, M. J. & Dugger, D. (1985, September). Effects of imipramine on depression and on obsessive-compulsive symptoms. Paper presented at the European Association for Behavior Therapy, Munich, West Germany.

Foa, E. B., Steketee, G. & Milby, J. B. (1980). Differential effects of exposure and response prevention in obsessive-compulsive washers. *Journal of Consulting and Clinical Psychology*, *48*, 71-79.

Foa, E. B., Steketee, G. & Ozarow, B. J. (1985). Behavior therapy with obsessive-compulsives: From theory to treatment. In M. Mavissakalian (Ed.), *Psychological and pharmacological treatments*. New York: Plenum.

Foa, E. B., Steketee, G., Turner, R. M. & Fisher, S. C. (1980). Effects of imaginal exposure to feared disasters in obsessive-compulsive checkers. *Behaviour Research and Therapy*, *18*, 449-455.

Gelder, M. G., Marks, I. M. & Wolff, H. H. (1967). Desensitization and psychotherapy in the treatment of phobic states: A controlled inquiry. *British Journal of Psychiatry*, *113*, 53-73.

Grayson, J. B., Foa, E. B. & Steketee, G. (1982). Habituation during exposure treatment: Distraction versus attention-focusing. *Behaviour Research and Therapy*, *20*, 323-328.

Grimshaw, L. (1965). The outcome of obsessional disorder, a follow-up study of 100 cases. *British Journal of Psychiatry*, *111*, 1051-1056.

Hafner, R. J. (1982). Marital interaction in persisting obsessive-compulsive disorders. *Australian and New Zealand Journal of Psychiatry*, *16*, 171-178.

Hudson, B. L. (1974). The families of agoraphobics treated by behaviour therapy. *British Journal of Social Work*, *4*, 51-59.

Ingram, I. M. (1961). Obsessional illness in mental hospital patients. *Journal of Mental Science*, *107*, 382-402.

Kringlen, E. (1965). Obsessional neurotics, a long term follow-up. *British Journal of Psychiatry*, *111*, 709-722.

Kringlen, E. (1970). Natural history of obsessional neuroses. *Seminars in Psychiatry*, *2*, 403-419.

Lang, P. J. (1979). A bio-informational theory of emotional imagery. *Psychophysiology*, *16*(6), 495-511.

Marks, I. M., Hodgson, R. & Rachman, S. (1975). Treatment of chronic obsessive-compulsives by *in vivo* exposure: A two year follow-up and issues in treatment. *British Journal of Psychiatry, 127*, 349-364.

Marks, I. M., Stern, R. S., Mawson, D., Cobb, J. & McDonald, R. (1980). Clomipramine and exposure for obsessive-compulsive rituals. *British Journal of Psychiatry, 136*, 1-25.

Mavissakalian, M., Turner, S. M., Michelson, L. & Jacob, R. (1985). Tricyclic antidepressants in obsessive-compulsive disorder: Antiobsessional or antidepressant agents? *American Journal of Psychiatry, 142*, 572-576.

Mawson, D., Marks, I. M. & Ramm, L. (1982). Clomipramine and exposure for chronic obsessive-compulsive rituals: Two year follow-up and further findings. *British Journal of Psychiatry, 140*, 11-18.

Meyer, V., Levy, R. & Schnurer, A. (1974). The behavioral treatment of obsessive-compulsive disorders. In H. R. Beech (Ed.), *Obsessional states*. London: Methuen.

Mills, H. L., Agras, W. S., Barlow, D. H. & Mills, J. R. (1973). Compulsive rituals treated by response prevention. *Archives of General Psychiatry, 28*, 524-527.

Nunes, J. S. & Marks, I. M. (1975). Feedback of true heart rate during exposure *in vivo*. *Archives of General Psychiatry, 32*, 933-996.

Pollack, J. M. (1979). Obsessive-compulsive personality: A review. *Psychological Bulletin, 86*, 225-241.

Rabavilas, A. D., Boulougouris, J. C. & Perissaki, C. (1979). Therapist qualities related to outcome with exposure *in vivo* in neurotic patients. *Journal of Behavior Therapy and Experimental Psychiatry, 10*, 293-299.

Rabavilas, A. D., Boulougouris, J. C. & Stefanis, C. (1976). Duration of flooding sessions in the treatment of obsessive-compulsive patients. *Behaviour Research and Therapy, 14*, 349-355.

Rachman, S. (1983). The modification of an agoraphobic avoidance behaviour: Some fresh possibilities. *Behaviour Research and Therapy, 21*, 567-574.

Rachman, S. J. & De Silva, P. (1978). Abnormal and normal obsessions. *Behaviour Research and Therapy, 16*, 233-248.

Rachman, S. & Hodgson, R. J. (1980). *Obsessions and compulsions*. Englewood Cliffs, NJ: Prentice Hall.

Rachman, S., Hodgson, R. & Marks, I. M. (1971). The treatment of chronic obsessive-compulsive neurosis. *Behaviour Research and Therapy, 9*, 237-247.

Rachman, S., Marks, I. & Hodgson, R. (1973). The treatment of obsessive-compulsive neurotics by modelling and flooding *in vivo*. *Behaviour Research and Therapy, 11*, 463-471.

Robertson, J., Wendiggersen, P. & Kaplan, I. (1983). Towards a comprehensive treatment for obsessional thoughts. *Behaviour Research and Therapy, 21*, 347-356.

Rosenberg, C. M. (1967). Personality and obsessional neurosis. *British Journal of Psychiatry, 113*, 471-477.

Salkovskis, P. M. & Harrison, J. (1984). Abnormal and normal obsessions: A replication. *Behaviour Research and Therapy, 22*, 549-552.

Salkovskis, P. M. & Warwick, H. M. C. (1985). Cognitive therapy of obsessive-compulsive disorder: Treating treatment failures. *Behavioral Psychotherapy, 13*, 243-255.

Sank, L. (1976). Counter-conditioning for a flight phobia. *Social Work, 21*, 318-319.

Schwartz, V. (1982). Prognostische kriterion bei der stationaren gruppen psychotherapie neurotisch depressiver und zwang a neurotisher patienten. *Zschr. Psychosom. Med., 28*, 30-51.

Slade, P. D. (1974). Psychometric studies of obsessional illness and obsessional personality. In H. R. Beech (Ed.), *Obsessional states*. London: Methuen.
Steiner, M., Welber, A., Archer, R. & Carrol, B. (1980). Multi-modal treatment of a
case of obsessive-compulsive neurosis. *Journal of Nervous and Mental Disorders,
168*, 184-187.
Steketee, G. & Foa, E. B. (1985). Behavioral treatment of obsessive-compulsive disorder: A guide for practice. In D. H. Barlow (Ed.), *Behavioral treatment of adult
disorders*. New York: Guilford Press.
Steketee, G., Foa, E. B. & Grayson, J. B. (1982). Recent advances in the behavioral
treatment of obsessive-compulsives. *Archives of General Psychiatry, 39*, 1365-
1371.
Steketee, G., Foa, E. B. & Kozak, M. J. (1985, September). Predictors of outcome for
obsessive-compulsives treated with exposure and response prevention. Presented at
the European Association for Behavior Therapy. Munich, West Germany.
Thyer, B. A. (1981). Prolonged *in vivo* exposure with a 70-year-old woman. *Journal of
Behavior Therapy and Experimental Psychiatry, 12*, 69-72.
Thyer, B. A. (1983). Behavior modification in social work practice. In M. Hersen, R.
M. Eisler & P. M. Miller (Eds.), *Progress in behavior modification*. New York:
Academic Press.
Traux, C. B. & Carkhuff, R. R. (1967). *Toward effective counseling in psychotherapy:
Training and practice*. Chicago: Aldine.
Turner, S. M., Hersen, M., Bellack, A. S., Andrasik, F. & Capparell, H. V. (1980).
Behavioral and pharmacological treatment of obsessive-compulsive disorders. *Jour-
nal of Nervous and Mental Disease, 168*, 651-657.
Turner, S. M., Hersen, M., Bellack, A. S. & Wells, K. C. (1970). Behavioral treat-
ment of obsessive-compulsive neurosis. *Behaviour Research and Therapy, 17*, 95-
106.
Wodarski, J. & Bagarozzi, D. (1979). *Behavioral social work*. New York: Human
Sciences Press.

Life Skills Counseling
for Preventing Problems
in Adolescence

Lewayne D. Gilchrist
Steven Paul Schinke
Josie Solseng Maxwell

SUMMARY. Many social and health problems first appear in adolescence. Prevention is a humane and cost effective approach for human services professionals who work with young people. This paper addresses theoretical, methodological, and outcome issues for the behavioral approach called life skills counseling for helping adolescents avoid potentially serious social and health problems. The authors define life skills, discuss the applicability of the life skills approach to problem prevention, provide an overview of life skills counseling methods, and present results from four applications of the life skills approach to preventing problems encountered in social work with adolescents.

Many social and health problems appear for the first time in adolescence. The period of life called adolescence encompasses more change than any other period in the life cycle.

The second decade of life is typically characterized by rapid physical and psychological development and a shift in the focus of influence from the family to peers. It is also a time of experimentation with alcohol, drugs, sex, and independence from adult authority. (Mechanic, 1983, p. 4)

The authors thank Sunnie Tasanasanta, Jill Brown, and Jean C. Seyfried. Funding was provided by the William T. Grant Foundation, National Institute on Drug Abuse DA03277, and National Cancer Institute CA29640. Requests for reprints should be sent to Lewayne D. Gilchrist, School of Social Work JH-30, University of Washington, Seattle, Washington 98195.

Substantial numbers of youth are seen by social workers and other human services professionals for such problems as school failure, substance abuse, accidents due to exceptional risk-taking, unplanned pregnancy, depression, and attempted suicide. Less visible but more prevalent are problems related to negotiating the normative tasks of adolescence — redefining relationships with parents and peers; finding, getting, and keeping a job; planning an adult vocation; and beginning to date.

This paper addresses theoretical, methodological, and outcome issues for the behavioral approach called life skills counseling for helping young people reduce or avoid problems in adolescence. The authors define life skills, discuss the applicability of the life skills approach to problem prevention, and provide an overview of life skills counseling methods. Finally, the authors illustrate the approach with applications of life skills methods to four problems encountered in social work with youth and adolescents. These problems are precocious sexual experimentation and risk of unintended pregnancy, drug and alcohol use, habitual cigarette smoking, and stress and social isolation in teenage mothers.

LIFE SKILLS

Prevention theorists have criticized human services professionals' near exclusive focus on identifying and eliminating pathology. More flexible, cost effective, and enduring clinical approaches appear to be those based on empowerment models aimed at promoting individual competence (Felner, Jason, Moritsugu & Farber, 1983; 1981). New clinical models therefore emphasize strengthening the fit between individuals and their environments through enhancing individuals' skills for dealing with environmental demands (cf. Germain & Gitterman, 1980; Lerner, Baker & Lerner, 1985; Meyer, 1983).

The capacity to respond successfully to environmental demands and to monitor and self-control transactions with the environment consists of a set of cognitive and behavioral skills. Such skills maximize individuals' chances for obtaining positive reinforcement from their environment while minimizing costs to themselves and others (Gilchrist, 1981). Naturally occurring reinforcement from the environment enhances individuals' sense of self-efficacy and self-esteem and thus reduces their need to engage in anti-social or risk taking behavior to gain respect from self and others. Skills for achieving this goal can be tailored and applied to a broad range of settings and circumstances across the life span and thus are defined as life skills. Life skills include the ability to solve problems, to communicate honestly and directly, to gain and maintain social support, and to control emotions and personal feelings. With the onset of adolescence, youth face significant shifts in school environments, role requirements, and social expectations. Lack of skills for smoothing these important transitions can lead to psychological discomfort strong enough to produce maladaptive and deviant behavior with serious and lasting consequences (Schinke & Gilchrist, 1984).

LIFE SKILLS AND PROBLEM PREVENTION

Most adolescents acquire many life skills through normal socialization. Discrete life skills, all of which ultimately increase adolescents' sense of self-efficacy, include the ability to disagree and to refuse, to relax and to contain distress within tolerable limits, to make requests, to plan, to initiate behavior, to disclose feelings, to anticipate the consequences of actions, and to accurately weigh pros and cons to make responsible decisions. These crucial skills allow adolescents to make and preserve interpersonal relationships, to cope with a constantly changing environmental context, and, in the end, to gain and maintain self-esteem.

But socialization processes are often incomplete. For some youth, critical skills are never acquired or are acquired too late to prevent serious social and health consequences. Cigarette smoking offers a health-related example of this problem generation process. A great many youth experiment with smoking in order to gain highly prized peer acceptance (Biglan et al., 1984). When cigarettes substitute for or replace the development of social and life skills and other means for achieving acceptance, youth can find themselves first psychologically, then physiologically addicted to tobacco and unintentionally launched on a lifetime of habitual smoking.

Recent data confirm that cigarette smoking is one of many problem behaviors in adolescence that is negatively correlated with social and other life skills (Gilchrist et al., 1985). Enhancing life skills thus appears a viable strategy for reducing youths' need to smoke and to engage in other problem behaviors. Within this model, problem prevention is achieved by providing adolescents with positive means (skills) for managing new social, psychological, and interpersonal demands in advance of youths' specific need for such skills.

LIFE SKILLS COUNSELING

In recent applications, life skills counseling programs have strengthened existing and introduced new skills to adolescents in three phases: cognitive preparation, skills acquisition, and practice of skills under less and less controlled circumstances. The cognitive preparation phase gives youth a persuasive rationale and motivation for participating in the program. The skills acquisition phase draws upon considerable research demonstrating the effectiveness of behavioral methods for initiating behavior change (cf. Bandura, 1977; Bellack & Hersen, 1979; Kendall & Hollon, 1979; Meichenbaum & Jaremko, 1983; Meyers & Craighead, 1984). The experiential practice phase provides exercises of increasing complexity to help youth generalize life skills to a variety of situations and to maintain this generalization over time (Schinke & Gilchrist, 1984).

The following sections outline methods and results from applications of the life skills counseling approach to reducing or preventing four problems encountered in social work with adolescents.

APPLICATIONS

Preventing Unintended Pregnancy

American adolescents begin experimenting with sexual behavior at earlier ages than ever before. By age 16, the majority of adolescents have had sexual intercourse (Baldwin, 1981). Most youth do not use contraception at first intercourse (Zelnik &

Shah, 1983). Many are sexually active for a year or more before investigating birth control. Not surprisingly, U.S. rates of unwanted adolescent pregnancy and childbearing are among the highest in the world (Wulf & Lincoln, 1985).

Several studies have applied the life skills approach to helping adolescents with sexual behavior and use of birth control (Gilchrist & Schinke, 1983, 1986; Schinke, Blythe & Gilchrist, 1981). In one such application, the life skills counseling approach was tested with 107 adolescents (61% male; mean age = 15.65 years) in a large public high school (Gilchrist & Schinke, 1983). After obtaining consent to participate, subjects were randomly assigned by classrooms to experimental and control conditions. All subjects were followed for 6 months.

Methods. The counseling program's cognitive preparation phase focused on sexual myths, the purpose and qualities of intimate relationships, and the translation of abstract facts about human reproduction into personal terms. The skills acquisition phase introduced a paradigm for generating multiple potential solutions to situations involving sexual decision making and sexual behavior. Skills were introduced for initiating and maintaining discussions of birth control in the face of partner opposition, disclosing feelings and opinions, and making requests and refusals. The skills practice phase involved role playing in small groups, covert rehearsal of skills using an imaginary partner, and completing behavioral homework assignments outside of the group counseling sessions. Assignments included pricing condoms in local drug stores and visiting Planned Parenthood and family planning clinics to pick up informational brochures.

Results. Analysis of videotaped performance tests indicated that at posttest, life skills condition subjects engaged in more effective problem solving, and had better communication skills when compared with control condition subjects. Life skills subjects also felt less anxious and more efficacious in handling situations involving sexual behavior. Follow-up data 6 months after the end of the life skills group sessions favored life skills over control condition subjects. Specifically, life skills subjects had better attitudes toward contraception, fewer instances of unprotected intercourse, greater protection at last intercourse, and less reliance on inadequate contraceptive methods. All differences noted between conditions were significant at less than the .05 level.

Stress and Social Isolation in Adolescent Mothers

Every year, over 600,000 babies are born to adolescents (The Alan Guttmacher Institute, 1981). Pregnancy and parenthood in adolescence involve significant and often abrupt social and role transitions. For many young mothers, such major and unanticipated life changes are accompanied by stress and isolation from former friends, activities, and sources of social support. Life skills counseling has been evaluated as a strategy for preventing stress and depression and improving mental health among young, unmarried adolescent mothers (Barth & Maxwell, 1985; Barth & Schinke, 1984).

One adaptation of life skills counseling to the special needs of young, unmarried parents involved 79 teenage mothers and mothers-to-be (Barth, Schinke & Maxwell, 1985). Most participants were Black (48%) or of other minority background (22%). Subjects gave their informed consent, obtained parental consent, and were pretested. A randomly selected one-half of the subjects participated in ten life skills group counseling sessions. All subjects were posttested, then followed for 4 months.

Methods. The cognitive preparation phase emphasized how mothers improve their child's self-esteem and life chances by improving their own. Counselors presented information on stress management with films and examples. The skills acquisition phase emphasized problem solving on issues common to young, low income parents — childrearing, job hunting, locating daycare, managing time, and handling money. Counselors demonstrated self-instruction skills to help subjects apply skills, accept limits, request aid, fend off criticism, and combat depression. In the skills practice phase, subjects completed homework to self-praise their daily accomplishments. In small groups, they rehearsed communication skills related to asking for help, refusing unwanted demands, and dealing with unwelcome advice.

Results. Analyses of posttest differences revealed greater improvements for life skills condition subjects than for control condition subjects on measures of conflict management and assertiveness. At posttest and follow-up, in contrast to control condition subjects, life skills condition subjects reported more supportive interactions with family members, friends, and male partners. For subjects who were mothers, parenting competence at follow-up improved in the life skills condition when compared with the control condition.

Smoking

Although smoking rates are beginning to fall for all age groups in this country, a significant number of adolescents every year still make the transition from experimenter to habitual smoker. Rates for smokeless tobacco use are rising precipitously for 10- to 18-year-olds. Life skills counseling has been applied to prevent smoking in adolescence (Gilchrist & Schinke, 1984, 1985; Gilchrist et al., 1986; Schinke & Gilchrist, 1984; Schinke, Gilchrist & Snow, 1985).

One evaluation of life skills counseling methods for preventing smoking involved 689 public school sixth graders (Schinke, Gilchrist & Snow, 1985). Once they consented and obtained parental consent, subjects were pretested and divided into life skills, information-only, and control conditions. Subjects in classrooms assigned to the life skills condition participated in ten, one-hour group sessions led by two social workers. Subjects assigned to the information-only condition participated in ten one-hour group sessions that involved discussion and opinion giving but no skills acquisition or practice. Control condition subjects participated in measurement only. All youths were posttested and followed for two years.

Methods. In the cognitive preparation phase, the life skills counselors emphasized subjects' coming transition into junior high and middle school. The life skills counselors showed subjects how inter- and intrapersonal pressures can lead to unplanned and undesirable behavior. Counselors discussed the advantages of possessing skills for managing situations that confront junior high school students. Peer pressure to smoke was presented as an example of one such situation.

The skills acquisition phase emphasized a problem-solving paradigm called SODAS for making good decisions in uncomfortable and uncertain circumstances. Communication skills were introduced by videotapes of youths who, first clumsily, then competently, responded to smoking-related peer pressure. The skills practice phase involved extensive small group role plays. During these practice sessions youths took turns as role players, coaches, and feedback sources.

Results. Analysis of covariance showed that at posttest, adolescents in the information-only condition were as knowledgeable about smoking as the life skills subjects and were more knowledgeable than control subjects. However, at 2-year follow-up life skills condition subjects reported the fewest intentions to smoke in the future and significantly lower rates of smoking. Both of these comparisons were significant at better than the .01 level. Self-reports of smoking were supplemented with biochemical measures. All subjects gave saliva samples which were analyzed for the smoking by-product, thiocyanate. At all follow-up periods, measures of cigarettes smoked in the past week significantly favored life skills condition subjects over information-only and control condition subjects.

Drug and Alcohol Use

Drug and alcohol use can be serious problems for many young people. Few subgroups have higher rates of substance use than American Indian youth (Trimble, 1984). Life skills counseling methods have been applied cross-culturally to help Indian adolescents avoid drug and alcohol use (Bobo, 1985; Schinke et al., 1985).

Culturally tailored life skills counseling methods were evaluated with 102 American Indian youths (51% male, *M* age = 11.34 years) (Gilchrist et al., in press). After subjects and their parents gave written consent, subjects were pretested, then randomly assigned to prevention or to test-only control conditions. Life skills condition subjects received 12 group counseling sessions from two American Indian social workers. All youths were posttested and followed for 6 months.

Methods. In the cognitive preparation phase, older Indian youths provided a rationale for the program by explaining why drug abuse is dissonant with the Indian Way, how substance use disserves the tribe and all Indian people, and how others have advanced their lives by not abusing drugs. The skills building phase introduced problem solving exercises to teach subjects to "think like elders" to see that opportunities to use drugs can be anticipated and avoided. Subjects said aloud, then silently practiced, self-instructional skills for controlling feelings and social pressures that lead to drug use. Because Indian youth are reticent to speak up in groups, the skills practice phase allowed subjects to operate stick puppets from behind screens to rehearse culturally appropriate communication skills. These practice sessions were accompanied by feedback, suggestions, and praise from leaders.

Results. From pretest to posttest, compared with control subjects, life skills condition subjects demonstrated more direct and indirect refusals of drugs and alcohol. Life skills subjects also reported less discomfort when refusing to participate in drug-related interactions. From pretest to 6-month follow-up, rates for tobacco and inhalant use did not differ. However, life skills condition subjects had lower rates of marijuana use and alcohol use when compared with control subjects. Most of these comparisons are significant at less than the .01 level.

DISCUSSION

Life skills counseling is a flexible clinical strategy with particular relevance for problem prevention in adolescence. The approach has been successfully tested with several adolescent populations addressing a variety of social and health problems with good results. In research to date, life skills methods have proven acceptable and attractive to adolescents, parents, school administrators, and community members. The rationale for life skills counseling is straightforward and easy to understand. The life skills counseling approach thus offers behavioral social workers guidelines for marketing as well as implementing effective prevention programs.

Like other behavioral approaches, life skills counseling rests on counselors' ability to provide accurate information and feedback to youth regarding effective behavior in a vast array of special settings and circumstances. A potential limitation of life skills counseling is lack of knowledge that may hinder professionals' ability to select and teach skills that are most salient for a particular individual, problem, or environmental setting. More research is needed on skills assessment techniques that are sensitive to adolescent development and to social norms impacting adolescents. Accurate assessment information is particularly critical for cross-cultural life skills counseling. More research is necessary to document assessment and intervention methods useful with young people from other ethnic and cultural minority groups.

There are limits to the applicability of the life skills approach. Although life skills counseling is a useful clinical tool, life skills methods cannot prevent problems rooted in racial discrimination or chronic poverty. In common with all behavioral technologies, life skills counseling methods must be combined with activities for achieving social and political change for disenfranchised young people.

With this caveat, the preventive potential of the approach remains. Many problems in adolescence can be anticipated because they are associated with developmental milestones and transitions common to all adolescents. Such predictable problems include stresses related to school transitions, to uneven physical growth and the onset of puberty, to entry into jobs and dating, and to changing patterns of family interaction as adolescents grow more independent. It may be that all young people can profit from life skills counseling focused on these common concerns. For some youth, adolescence is additionally complicated because of unexpected changes and life crises such as parental divorce or unintended pregnancy. The life skills approach also appears appropriate for reducing and preventing problems experienced by these special high risk adolescent groups. The approach deserves further evaluation in these and other contexts.

REFERENCES

The Alan Guttmacher Institute (1981). *Teenage pregnancy: The problem that hasn't gone away*. New York: The Alan Guttmacher Institute.

Baldwin, W. H. (1981). Adolescent pregnancy and childbearing—An overview. *Seminars in Perinatology, 5*, 1-8.

Bandura, A. (1977). *Social learning theory*. Englewood Cliffs, NJ: Prentice-Hall.

Barth, R. & Maxwell, J. S. (1985). Preventing depression and dysfunction among adolescent mothers. In L. D. Gilchrist & S. P. Schinke (Eds.), *Preventing social and health problems through life skills training.* Seattle: Center for Social Welfare Research, Monograph #3, University of Washington.

Barth, R. & Schinke, S. P. (1984). Enhancing the social supports of teenage mothers. *Social Casework, 65,* 523-531.

Barth, R. P., Schinke, S. P. & Maxwell, J. S. (1985). Coping skills training for school-age mothers. *Journal of Social Service Research, 8,* 75-94.

Bellack, A. S. & Hersen, M. (Eds.) (1979). *Research and practice in social skills training.* New York: Plenum.

Biglan, A., McConnell, S., Severson, H. H., Bavry, J. & Ary D. (1984). A situational analysis of adolescent smoking. *Journal of Behavioral Medicine, 9,* 109-122.

Bobo, J. K. (1985). Preventing drug abuse among American Indian adolescents. In L. D. Gilchrist & S. P. Schinke (Eds.), *Preventing social and health problems through life skills training.* Seattle: Center for Social Welfare Research, Monograph #3, University of Washington.

Felner, R. D., Jason, L. A., Moritsugu, J. N. & Farber, S. S. (1983). *Preventive psychology: Theory, research, and practice.* New York: Pergamon.

Germain, C. B. & Gitterman, A. (1980). *The life model of social work practice.* New York: Columbia University.

Gilchrist, L. D. (1981). Social competence in adolescence. In S. P. Schinke (Ed.), *Behavioral methods in social welfare,* pp. 61-80. New York: Aldine.

Gilchrist, L. D. & Schinke, S. P. (1983). Coping with contraception: Cognitive and behavioral methods with adolescents. *Cognitive Therapy and Research, 7,* 379-388.

Gilchrist, L. D., & Schinke, S. P. (1984). Self-control skills for smoking prevention. In P. F. Engstrom, P. N. Anderson & L. E. Mortensen (Eds.), *Advances in cancer control: 1983,* pp. 125-130. New York: Alan R. Liss.

Gilchrist, L. D. & Schinke, S. P. (1985). Improving smoking prevention programs. *Journal of Psychosocial Oncology, 3,* 67-78.

Gilchrist, L. D. & Schinke, S. P. (1986). Increasing sexual and contraceptive responsibility. In A. R. Stiffman & R. A. Feldman (Eds.), *Advances in adolescent mental health: Treatment methods and issues, Vol. 2* (pp. 27-36). Greenwich, CT: JAI.

Gilchrist, L. D., Schinke, S. P., Bobo, J. K. & Snow, W. P. (in press). Self-control skills for preventing smoking. *Addictive Behaviors, 11,* 169-174.

Gilchrist, L. D., Schinke, S. P., Bobo, J. K., Trimble, J. E. & Cvetkovich, G. T. (in press). Skills enhancement to prevent substance abuse among American Indian adolescents. *International Journal of the Addictions.*

Gilchrist, L. D., Snow, W. H., Lodish, D. & Schinke, S. P. (1985). The relationship of cognitive and behavioral skills to adolescent tobacco smoking. *Journal of School Health, 55,* 132-134.

Kendall, P. C. & Hollon, S. D. (1979). *Cognitive-behavioral interventions.* New York: Academic.

Lerner, J. V., Baker, N. & Lerner, R. M. (1985). A person-context goodness of fit model of adjustment. *Advances in Cognitive-Behavioral Research and Therapy, 4,* 111-136.

Mechanic, D. (1983). Adolescent health and illness behavior: Review of the literature and a new hypothesis for the study of stress. *Journal of Human Stress, 9,* 4-13.

Meichenbaum, D. & Jaremko, M. E. (Eds.) (1983). *Stress reduction and prevention.* New York: Plenum.

Meyer, C. H. (1983). *Clinical social work in the eco-systems perspective.* New York: Columbia University.

Meyers, A. W. & Craighead, W. E. (1984). *Cognitive behavior therapy with children.* New York: Plenum.

Schinke, S. P., Blythe, B. J. & Gilchrist, L. D. (1981). Brief reports: Cognitive-behavioral prevention of adolescent pregnancy. *Journal of Counseling Psychology, 28,* 451-454.

Schinke, S. P. & Gilchrist, L. D. (1984). Preventing cigarette smoking with youth. *Journal of Primary Prevention, 5*(1), 48-56.

Schinke, S. P., Gilchrist, L. D. & Snow, W. H. (1985). Skills intervention to prevent cigarette smoking among adolescents. *American Journal of Public Health, 75,* 665-666.

Schinke, S. P., Schilling, R. F., Gilchrist, L. D., Barth, R. P., Bobo, J. K., Trimble, J. E. & Cvetkovich, G. T. (1985). Preventing substance abuse with American Indian youth. *Social Casework, 66*(4), 213-217.

Trimble, J. E. (1984). Drug abuse prevention research needs among American Indians and Alaska Natives. *White Cloud Journal, 3,* 23-34.

Wulf, D. & Lincoln, R. (1985). Doing something about teenage pregnancy. *Family Planning Perspectives, 17,* 52.

Zelnik, M. & Shah, F. K. (1983). First intercourse among young Americans. *Family Planning Perspectives, 15,* 64-70.

Treatment Compliance
in Social Work

Rona L. Levy

SUMMARY. This paper provides an overview of the area of client compliance with treatment regimens. The definition of compliance and rationale for social work involvement in compliance research are presented. Recommendations for specific topics and methodological procedures for social work research are also discussed.

Beginning a decade ago (Levy & Carter, 1976; Levy, 1978),* social workers were encouraged to become aware of and involved in the investigation of patient compliance with treatment regimens. These recommendations have gone largely unheeded, even though this area is as, if not more, in need of good research as it was then. This paper will begin be defining compliance and addressing why client compliance is a critical area for social work clinical research. Several topics for compliance research will then be overviewed. These topics were chosen on the basis of research into the most effective methods to enhance client compliance. Specific suggestions for future research on each topic are presented. The concluding section highlights some of the methodological problems with compliance research and offers suggestions for alternative research strategies.

Health care is emphasized in this paper because many social workers are employed in health care settings. Nevertheless, clini-

---

Portions of this paper originally appeared in Shelton, J. L. and Levy, R. L. (1981). *Behavioral assignments and treatment compliance.* Champaign, Illinois: Research Press.

---

*None of us are modest, but it helps to give the appearance of it.

85

cal issues in other areas will be covered and it will also be easy to extrapolate from health care to more generic clinical practice.

DEFINITION OF COMPLIANCE

Compliance is what occurs when an assignment is carried out by the client in the way it was given by the assignment giver(s). Many social workers object to the term "compliance." The primary objection seems to be a dislike for the implication that a client complies with the dictates of the clinician, a situation which seems to run counter to the social work value of having the client actively involved in treatment. Alternative terms, such as "adherence" (to the treatment regimen) have been suggested to reduce this implication. Nevertheless, this concern is unfounded. The term compliance is consistent with much of the research literature and the definition of compliance here states "in the way [an assignment] was given *by the assignment giver*," not "by the clinician." Thus, clients alone or with the aid of clinicians may be the assignment givers. Compliance may be increased by involving clients in the assignment-giving process, as will be discussed later.

Why Study Compliance?

The position taken here and elsewhere is that client compliance is the *basis* of outpatient clinical practice, and especially clinical behavioral practice (Kanfer & Phillips, 1969; Shelton & Levy, 1981a). In the typical clinical situation, clients may be assessed, trained, or receive a variety of treatment procedures while in face-to-face contact with the therapist. But all this activity would be useless if the client did not follow certain procedures when away from this direct clinician contact, in her or his natural environment. Considering some of the topics in this special issue, how far would treatment progress if the adolescent did not practice new life skills with his or her peers, if the obsessive-compulsive did not rehearse alternative responses when in high-risk situations, if the spouses of alcoholics did not use new strategies with their spouses, or if parents did not appropriately apply management techniques with their children?

Health care is one area where patient compliance is critical. Increasingly over recent years, health care workers have realized that the development of new medicines and medical procedures alone will not significantly alter the health of individuals in our society. Rather, lifestyle or behavioral change will produce the greatest health benefit. Thus, we are encouraged to follow healthy diet and exercise patterns as well as eliminate such health risks as smoking. Even within traditional medical practice, patients must typically carry out a large portion of their own treatment. They may be asked to take medicines, monitor blood levels (as in the treatment of diabetes), conduct procedures as complex as self-hemodyalysis regimen or participate in a variety of other techniques on which the success of the treatment depends. A literature search on the topic of patient compliance will yield approximately 70 new articles each month, attesting to the emphasis on this topic in the medical literature. Unfortunately, almost none of these articles are directed at the social work audience.

Social work is missing a golden opportunity to render effective service. As will be discussed later, many of the most critical areas of investigation in compliance, such as social support, are appropriate for social workers who are already integrated into settings where compliance research would be easy to conduct. Finally, traditional health care providers in the federal government are very interested in encouraging work in this area. Physicians are most anxious to have trained social workers examine ways to alter their compliance problems with patients and a number of RFPs (requests for proposals) have been emerging from the federal government on this topic.

TOPICS FOR COMPLIANCE RESEARCH

Rates of Compliance

Many of the articles in the medical literature are simply studies of whether compliance occurs in a particular setting. The question of compliance rates has been almost virtually ignored in behavior therapy and social work. This is particularly troublesome since the experience from medicine is that noncompliance rates are often exceedingly high (Haynes, Taylor & Sackett, 1979). Shelton and Levy (1979, 1981b) report that while a majority of treatment studies in the behavior therapy literature rely on client practice of assignments, only seven percent of the articles reported actual compliance rates. These data were based on a survey of all treatment articles published over a six-year period in eight leading behavior therapy journals. The authors outline several advantages which would be derived from researchers providing data on compliance in their research reports:

> First, if noncompliance occurs and is related to adverse case outcomes, clinicians and researchers could alter their own behavior to address this problem. If noncompliance occurs, but is not related to case outcome, ineffective components of treatment (such as some assignments) could be eliminated. Furthermore, readers provided with information on homework and compliance would be better able to evaluate treatment methods and, if desired, more accurately replicate these methods. (1981b, p. 14)

Compliance-Enhancement Strategies

Several methods for enhancing compliance have been studied by both correlational and hypothesis-testing research. This section will review much of the previous work and suggest directions for future research.

The specificity of assignments. A substantial amount of research on compliance with instructions supports the notion that specific instructions are more likely to be followed than those that are less specific (Doster, 1972; Kanfer, Karoly & Newman, 1974; Liebert, Hanratty & Hill, 1969; Rappaport, Gross & Lepper, 1973; Svarstad, 1976). The success of contracting procedures (Steckel & Swain, 1977) may also be taken as evidence of the value of explicitness. To meet all contingencies, contracts require clear and specific descriptions of the required behaviors.

It must be remembered, however, that specificity should not result in making the behavior too complex or too difficult. Haynes et al. (1979) note that more complex and demanding prescriptions are met with greater noncompliance. This is also supported by the research on concept formation (Flanders & Thistlethwaite, 1970). In short, simplicity should not be sacrificed in the search for specificity.

Future research might test the effect on compliance of several levels of specificity in giving an assignment. More research on the effectiveness of contracting procedures by social workers is also needed.

Direct skill training. A significant body of research has demonstrated that use of participant modeling and behavior rehearsal enhances learning behavior (Bandura, 1979; Lewis, 1974; McFall & Marston, 1970). Feedback and reinforcement during practice sessions may also augment the learning experience (Locke, Cartledge & Koeppel, 1968; Leitenberg, 1975). In medical programs, supervised practice of assigned tasks also has been used as a compliance enhancer (Bowen, Rich & Schlatfeldt, 1961).

Several papers in this special issue also discuss research on the effects of direct skill training, as well as point the way for future research in their respective areas.

Positive reinforcement. It is very likely unnecessary to mention to the audience of this special issue the potential effectiveness of positive reinforcement to increase the occurrence of a behavior which it follows, including compliance. Nevertheless, some examples will be covered here. In the medical literature, Mahoney, Moura, and Wade (1973) found that positive reinforcement had more effect than other strategies in their program, and Agras, Barlow, Chapin, Abel and Leitenberg (1974) showed the power of positive reinforcement in the treatment of anorexia nervosa. The use of written contracts in obesity treatment also demonstrate the effects of positive reinforcement in enhancing compliance (Harris & Bruner, 1971; Leon, 1976; Mann, 1972).

Many studies (Becker & Green, 1975; Blackwell, 1979; Brownlee, 1978; Christensen, 1978; Stokols, 1975; Stuart & Davis, 1972) report that mediators from the client's natural environment are important in both monitoring (which will be discussed later) and delivering positive reinforcement. Use of mediators from the natural environment may be one way of operationalizing "social support." Social workers are often the persons most familiar with a client's social support system and would thus be in an excellent position to identify and work with these individuals.

In two reports of hypothesis-testing research on a weight reduction program and its follow-up results, Israel and Saccone
(1979) and Saccone and Israel (1978) found that monetary reinforcement by spouses was the most effective incentive for producing and maintaining weight loss. Zitter and Freemouw (1978)
investigated whether individuals complied more when they themselves received a reward, or when they saw that someone else
suffered by their noncompliance. In this experiment, subjects in
one group lost money if their partner did not lose weight. Partners were friends chosen by the clients. Interestingly, the part-
ner-consequated condition was less effective. The authors suggest that partners may have reinforced client noncompliance.

Environmental mediators have been used in several nonobesity
programs as well. Dapcich-Miura and Hovell (1979) used a multiple baseline-reversal single-subject experimental design to
demonstrate that a token reinforcement contingency administered
by a subject's granddaughter could be used to increase juice and
medication consumption and walking. Tokens were redeemable
for the subject's dinner selection. Lowe and Lutzker (1979) also
used a multiple baseline design to demonstrate that a point system with backup reinforcers could be effective in motivating a
nine-year-old female diabetic to comply with dieting, urine-test-
ing, and foot-care regimens. The child's mother both monitored
compliance and delivered prompts and reinforcement.

Further research should continue to investigate the effects of
various types of reinforcers given by various sources across a
range of social work clinical settings.

Shaping assignment giving. Techniques of minimal initial demands that gradually increase over time have found some support
in the literature on attitude change, and some experiments have
strongly supported the effectiveness of the "foot-in-the-door"
effect. In two experiments, Freedman and Fraser (1966) showed
that suburban housewives were more likely to submit to a major
request (such as allowing a large unattractive billboard to be
placed on their front lawn, or allowing a survey team to enter
their homes and catalog their household products) if they had
first complied with a simple request like signing an innocuous
petition, answering a few survey questions, or placing a sign in
their window supporting safe driving or a beautiful California. In

a later study, Lepper (1973) helped extend the generality of this effect in an experiment on the resistance to temptation of second-grade children. As predicted, children who resisted the temptation to play with an attractive toy under minimal-threat conditions tended to resist the temptation to cheat in a game played three weeks later more than children who were not exposed to the initial situation or who were exposed to it under high-threat conditions. Lepper stresses the importance of the initial compliance being obtained under relatively low demand conditions.

It is easy to conceptualize future studies where one group of clients are asked to do all of an assignment in some area and other groups are only asked to do their assignment in increasing increments. Groups could then be compared on which conditions eventually produced greater overall compliance rates.

Reminders. In studies in the medical literature, patients frequently report "forgetting" as a reason for noncompliance (Alpert, 1964; Badgley & Furnal, 1961; Harfouche, Abi-Yaghi, Melidossian & Azouri, 1973). Some experimental studies have tested the effects of reminders on appointment keeping. Shepard and Moseley (1976) and Gates and Colborn (1976) compared compliance rates for subjects who received mail or phone reminders to compliance rates for those who received no reminders. Both types of reminders significantly improved the appointment-keeping rates for experimental group subjects over the rates for subjects in the control condition.

Finer discriminations on the type of cues and the effect of cuing over time have also been made. Nazarian, Machuber, Charney, and Coulter (1974) compared the effect of two types of reminder cards on appointment keeping. Both cards indicated the date and time of the appointment, and one card also noted the physician or nurse and the reason for the appointment. No difference in compliance was found when one or the other type of card was used. However, both groups receiving cards had a significantly higher appointment-keeping rate than the control group.

Also interesting was the indication that the reminders seemed to have a greater effect as the interval between appointments increased. The smallest appointment interval in this study was 12 days. In addition, the study by Levy and Claravell (1977) tested the effect of reminders on patients with between-appointment intervals of as low as three days. Such studies show it is possible to compare the effect of reminders with a wide range of interval periods. In the Levy and Claravell study, reminders had a significant effect on patients whose appointments were more than two weeks apart, but no significant effect on patients whose appointments were scheduled within a two-week period.

Further research is needed on the many parameters that will influence the effectiveness of a cue on compliance. For example, we do not know the optimal interval from delivery of a reminder to expected compliance, or how the content of a reminder could influence compliance. Some studies have failed to show that reminders enhance appointment-keeping rates (Barkin & Duncan, 1975; Kidd & Euphrat, 1971; Krause, 1966). In a review of this literature, Frankel and Hovell (1978) suggest that negative results may be due to variations in the clinics or in the selection of patients to be reminded (for example, Kidd and Euphrat, 1971, only looked at subjects who had previously failed).

Public commitment. The author conducted a series of experiments to test the effect of public commitment on compliance. In the first (Levy, 1977), clients in an outpatient behavior therapy setting were asked to phone the therapist in a few days to set up a subsequent appointment. Subjects randomly assigned to a "verbal commitment" experimental condition were given the assignment and asked if they would comply. In addition to asking for a verbal commitment (or a head nod) to indicate intended compliance, subjects randomly assigned to a second experimental condition — the "verbal and written commitment" group — were also asked to sign a form indicating that they would comply. Subjects in the control condition were merely given the assignment. Subjects complied more in the commitment conditions than the control condition, with the highest compliance rates in the verbal and written commitment condition. In a second study (Levy, Yamashita & Pow, 1979), patients reporting for a flu inoculation were asked to return a postcard within 48 hours to indicate whether they were experiencing any symptoms. Subjects randomly assigned to the experimental condition were asked to verbally (or by nodding) indicate their intention to comply. Again, experimental subjects returned more cards and at a faster rate than control subjects.

In a final study (Levy & Clark, 1980), however, the effect of a public commitment was not replicated. Subjects given a reappointment time and randomly placed in a commitment experimental or a no-commitment control condition were compared on appointment keeping rates. No differences between the experimental and control conditions were found.

Replicating the series of studies by Levy and her colleagues, Wurtele, Galanos, and Roberts (1980) also found that both verbal and verbal plus written commitment conditions were positively associated with compliance. Patient return rate for skintest reading during a TB detection drive was the major dependent variable.

This series seems to be weighted in favor of the positive effects of eliciting a public commitment from clients. Further research will be needed to specify the parameters — such as the type of assignment, the setting, and the client population — where this compliance enhancer is most effective.

Private commitments. The Health Belief Model, developed by Rosenstock (1966), outlines several areas of patient beliefs that are believed to be important in increasing compliance with medical regimens (Becker & Maiman, 1975; Maiman & Becker, 1974; Maiman, Becker, Kirscht, Haefner & Drachman, 1977). Several studies have demonstrated relationships between health beliefs and medical compliance, and much of this information would be useful for extrapolation to therapy situations. Included in health beliefs are perceptions about one's own sense of control, the priority one puts on health in one's life, the perceived severity of the illness, and the cues for action that are available to the client. Although several studies support the Health Belief Model, a large number have not found relationships between compliance and health beliefs (Haynes et al., 1979). Variation across situations may be a critical factor here.

Several writers in the behavior therapy literature have discussed the role of expectation in treatment (Wilson & Evans, 1972). Expectation, as these authors point out, may bridge the gap between present difficult tasks and ultimate success. It may also help clients to remain in treatment. Finally, treatment that is

inconsistent with a client's expectations of it may result in reduced compliance (Davis, 1968; Francis, Korsch & Morris,
1969).

Some studies have supported the value of client participation
in decision making. Kanfer and Grimm (1978) found that subjects who were given a choice of several behavioral methods designed to increase reading performance did significantly better
than those who had no choice. Lovitt and Curtiss (1969) found
that children showed higher rates of academic behaviors such as
studying when they were allowed to participate in their own
treatment plan. A similar study by Brigham and Bushell (1972)
revealed that children would work to earn control over their own
rewards. In this particular study, the authors found that individual response rates were higher even when the self-imposed reinforcement conditions were identical to those imposed by a
teacher. Likewise, Phillips (1966) demonstrated that clients who
helped in the design of their own treatment were more motivated
to change.

Schulman (1979) developed a measure of Active Patient Orientation (APO) that determined the extent to which patients perceived themselves to be "addressed as active participants, involved in therapeutic planning and equipped to carry out
self-care activities" (p. 278). High APO was associated with
greater blood pressure control, adherence, understanding, and
fewer medication errors. Since contracts, discussed earlier as a
tool for establishing a contingency relationship, may also be effective because they give patients an opportunity to discuss treatment options and participate in treatment decisions, it is not surprising that patients assigned to a contracting group in a larger
study showed higher APO scores.

Cognitive rehearsal. Several studies have shown the worth of
using cognitive rehearsal to improve targeted behaviors. In one
study Nesse and Nelson (1977) used between-session rehearsals
of covert modeling on cigarette smoking reduction. In covert
modeling the client was asked to imagine a competent model
engaging in the behaviors he or she wished to develop. In this
particular study subjects were asked to imagine themselves feeling an urge to smoke, making an alternative nonsmoking response, and then receiving a favorable consequence for not

smoking. Results showed that covert rehearsal combined with self-reinforcement was more effective than covert rehearsal alone in reducing cigarette smoking.

During the 12th Winter Olympics, Suinn (1977) worked with the athletes of the United States' cross-country skiing and biathalon teams. Suinn developed a package composed of his Visual Motor Behavior Rehearsal, thought stopping, and covert positive reinforcement to counteract pain sensations. The athletes' self-report indicated that this behavioral-cognitive treatment package improved their performance. Interestingly, one of the skiers won a silver medal, the first medal won by an American in Nordic racing. However, because of the lack of objective controls, the conclusions of this research should only be taken as suggestive.

Other studies have confirmed the importance of using covert rehearsal as a means of enhancing subject behaviors outside the therapeutic hour. For example, this technique has been shown to be effective in reducing fear (Cautela, Flannery & Hanley, 1974; Kazdin, 1973, 1974a, 1974b, 1974c), in increasing assertive behavior (Kazdin, 1974d, 1975, 1976a, 1976b), and in decreasing alcoholic and obsessive-compulsive behavior (Hay, Hay & Nelson, 1977). Research applying this technique to enhance compliance with homework in social work practice would be desirable.

Reduction of the negative effects of compliance. Social workers in medical settings traditionally have been involved in reducing the barriers to patient compliance with treatment regimens. If patients were asked to do such things as "stay off their feet" or "enter an outpatient treatment program," it is usually the social worker, often in the role of discharge planner, who works to facilitate these events.

Empirical support for the effectiveness of this compliance enhancer is found in reports discussing the effects of general social work intervention (Olson & Levy, 1981), which often do not isolate this specific compliance-enhancer component, as well as client self-reports of barriers to compliance. These barriers include finances, transportation, and unemployment. However, experimental data to support these reasons have not been convincing. For example, Sackett et al. found no increase in compliance by locating client treatment centers on the worksite as opposed to use of community-based treatment facilities (Sackett,

Haynes, Gibson, Hackett, Taylor, Roberts & Johnson, 1975). Further experimental work is needed to test their findings in a variety of settings with different patient populations.

Additional support for enhancing compliance by counteracting potential punishers derive from the almost self-evident position that punished behavior is likely to decrease, and a large number of studies support this position. Clients complain of punishment following assertive responses or cite side effects as another reason for noncompliance with medical regimens (Ballweg & McCorquodale, 1974; Caldwell et al., 1970). Exactly how much reinforcement, of what kind, and in what situations can offset punishment has yet to be investigated.

Monitoring. Monitoring has been used extensively as a component of successful treatment programs in several studies in both behavior therapy and medicine. Books by Ciminero, Calhoun, and Adams (1977), Cone and Hawkins (1977), Haynes (1978), Haynes and Wilson (1979), and Keefe, Kopel, and Gordon (1978), as well as the journals, *Behavioral Assessment* and the *Journal of Behavioral Assessment*, provide documentation of its use. For example, self-monitoring has been used in studies for taking medication (Carnahan & Nugent, 1975; Deberry, Jefferies & Light, 1975; Epstein & Masek, 1978; Haynes et al., 1976; Moulding, 1961) and in obesity treatment programs (Bellack, 1976; Kingsley & Shapiro, 1977).

Several examples of monitoring by others to enhance compliance have also been reported in both the behavior therapy and medical literature. Monitoring plus reinforcement by mediators has also been an effective component of several treatment programs (Brownlee, 1978; Stuart & Davis, 1972). Clinician monitoring of blood pressure has been a part of some strategies to enhance compliance with antihypertension regimens (McKenney, Slining, Henderson, Devins & Barr, 1973; Takala, Niemela, Rosti & Silvers, 1979). In addition, direct observation of desirable behaviors has been reported in the behavior therapy literature for eating (Epstein & Martin, 1977), drinking (Miller, 1978), and sexual behaviors (Zeiss, 1978), using colleagues, friends or relatives, and spouses, respectively. While many studies have incorporated monitoring into an intervention package or studied the effect of monitoring as an intervention itself, more research is needed on the implementation of monitoring to enhance compliance and the variables that influence the effects of monitoring on compliance.

METHODOLOGY FOR COMPLIANCE RESEARCH

Earlier writings have made several methodological suggestions which would increase the quality of compliance research (Levy, 1980, 1983, 1985, in press). While these suggestions primarily addressed research on the effects of social support on compliance, they are relevant to all areas of compliance research.

The Measurement of the Compliance Enhancer

Variables studied in compliance research must be effectively operationalized. Global terms such as "social support," which are defined differently across studies produce uninterpretable and inconsistent experimental findings. Operational definitions which rely on observable data provide better opportunities to assess reliability and validity than do other methods of assessment (Barlow, Hayes & Nelson, 1984). Furthermore, reliability and validity data should always be obtained and reported.

The Measurement of Compliance

As Gordis (1979) and others have cautioned, clinical outcome may be affected by a variety of factors other than compliance. Thus, researchers who study compliance should not rely solely on clinical outcome to determine if compliance has occurred. Specific, reliable, and valid measures of *compliance behavior* are far superior as outcome measures.

The Manipulation of the Compliance-Enhancement Variable

If an experiment is to allow valid conclusions about the effect of one variable upon another, then the manipulated variable must be introduced to subjects as the researcher plans and states it to be. As Johnston and Pennypacker note (1980):

The independent variable must be represented by some environmental event, the physical parameters of which are known, specified, and controlled to the extent required. Such a clear description of the independent variable is essential if any factually accurate statement is to issue from the experimental effort (p. 39).

Unfortunately, few precautions and little monitoring occur in the compliance research literature (along with research in other fields) to guarantee such integrity of the independent variable (Peterson, Homer & Wonderlich, 1982). For example, in one study where home visits were manipulated and their effect on compliance was measured, the authors state "it is not known how 'pure' the home visiting intervention was" (Earp, Ory & Strogatz, 1982, p. 1152).

Another study reports only "casual observation" to determine how the compliance-enhancing independent variable was manipulated (Caplan, Harrison, Wellins & French, 1980). Social work researchers must use more rigorous procedures, with as much attention being paid to their independent variables as to their dependent variables.

CONCLUSION

Compliance is critical to good behavioral social work practice. Little research has been conducted by social workers to find ways to enhance compliance with treatment regimens. Social workers should become more active in this area. If researchers investigate many of the unaddressed problems in the compliance literature and if they follow sound methodological procedures, significant contributions will result.

REFERENCES

Agras, W. S., Barlow, D. H. Chapin, H. N., Abel, G. C. & Leitenberg, H. (1974). Behavior modification of anorexia nervosa. *Archives of General Psychiatry, 30,* 279-286.

Alpert, J. J. (1964). Broken appointments. *Pediatrics, 34,* 127-132.

Badgley, R. F. & Furnal, M. A. (1961). Appointment breaking in a pediatric clinic. *Yale Journal of Biology and Medicine, 34,* 117-123.

Ballweg, J. A. & McCorquodale, D. W. (1974). Family planning method change and dropouts in the Phillippines. *Social Biology, 21*, 88-95.

Bandura, A. (1969). *Principles of behavior modification*. New York: Holt, Rinehart & Winston.

Barkin, R. M. & Duncan, R. (1975). Broken appointments: Questions, not answers. *Pediatrics, 55*, 747-748.

Barlow, D. H., Hayes, S. C. & Nelson, R. O. (1984). *The scientist practitioner*. New York: Pergamon.

Becker, M. H. & Green, L. W. (1975). A family approach to compliance with medical treatment. *International Journal of Health Education, 18*, 175-182.

Becker, M. H. & Maiman, L. A. (1975). Sociobehavioral determinants of compliance with health and medical care recommendations. *Medical Care, 13*, 10-24.

Bellack, A. S. (1976). A comparison of self-reinforcement and self-monitoring in a weight reduction program. *Behavior Therapy, 7*, 68-75.

Blackwell, B. (1979). Treatment adherence: A contemporary overview. *Psychosomatics, 20*, 27-35.

Bowen, R. G., Rich, R. & Schlatfeldt, R. M. (1961). Effects of organized instruction for patients with the diagnosis of diabetes mellitus. *Nursing Research, 10*, 151-155.

Brigham, G. & Bushell, D. (1972). Notes on autonomous environments: Student selected vs. teacher-selected rewards. Unpublished manuscript, University of Kansas.

Brownlee, A. (1978). The family and health care: Explorations in cross-cultural settings. *Social Work in Health Care, 4*, 179-198.

Caldwell, J. R., Cobb, S., Dowling, M. D. & DeJonhg, D. (1970). The dropout problem in antihypertensive therapy. *Journal of Chronic Diseases, 22*, 579-592.

Caplan, R. D., Harrison, R. V., Wellins, R. V. & French, J. R. P. (1980). *Social support and patient adherence: Experimental and survey findings*. Ann Arbor: Institute for Social Research.

Carnahan, J. E. & Nugent, C. A. (1975). The effects of self-monitoring by patients on the control of hypertension. *The American Journal of Medical Sciences, 269*, 69-73.

Cautela, J., Flannery, R. & Hanley, S. (1974). Covert modeling: An experimental test. *Behavior Therapy, 5*, 494-502.

Christensen, D. B. (1978). Drug-taking compliance: A review and synthesis. *Health Services Research, 13*, 171-187.

Ciminero, A. R., Calhoun, K. S. & Adams, H. E. (1977). *Handbook of behavioral assessment*. New York: John Wiley & Sons.

Cone, J. D. & Hawkins, R. P. (1977). *Behavioral assessment: New directions in clinical psychology*. New York: Brunner/Mazel.

Dapcich-Miura, E. & Hovell, M. F. (1979). Contingency management of adherence to a complex medical regimen in an elderly heart patient. *Behavior Therapy, 10*, 193-210.

Davis, M. S. (1968). Variations in patients compliance with doctors' advice: An empirical analysis of patterns of communication. *American Journal of Public Health, 58*, 274-288.

Deberry, P., Jefferies, L. P. & Light, M. R. (1975). Teaching cardiac patients to manage medications. *American Journal of Nursing, 75*, 2121-2193.

Doster, J. A. (1972). Effects of instructions, modeling and role rehearsal on interview verbal behavior. *Journal of Consulting and Clinical Psychology, 39*, 202-209.

Earp, J. L., Ory, M. G. & Strogatz, D. S. (1982). The effects of family involvement and practitioner home visits on the control of hypertension. *American Journal of Public Health, 72*, 1146-1154.

Epstein, L. H. & Martin, J. E. (1977). Compliance and side effects of weight reduction groups. *Behavior Modification, 11*, 551-558.

Epstein, L. H. & Masek, B. J. (1978). Behavioral control of medicine compliance. *Journal of Applied Behavior Analysis, 11*, 1-9.

Flanders, J. P. & Thistlethwaite, D. L. (1970). Effects of informative and justificatory variables upon imitation. *Journal of Experimental Social Psychology, 6*, 316-328.

Francis, V. F., Korsch, B. M. & Morris, M. (1969). Gaps in doctor-patient communication: Patients' response to medical advice. *New England Journal of Medicine, 280*, 535-540.

Frankel, B. S. & Hovell, M. F. (1978). Health service appointment keeping. *Behavior Modification, 2*, 435-464.

Freedman, J. L. & Fraser, S. C. (1966). Compliance without pressure: The foot-in-the-door technique. *Journal of Personality and Social Psychology, 4*, 195-202.

Gates, S. J. & Colborn, D. K. (1976). Lowering appointment failures in a neighborhood health center. *Medical Care, 14*, 263-267.

Gordis, L. (1979). Conceptual and methodologic problems in measuring patient compliance. In R. B. Haynes, D. W. Taylor & D. L. Sackett (Eds.), *Compliance in health care*, pp. 23-43. Baltimore: Johns Hopkins.

Harfouche, J., Abi-Yahgi, M., Melidossian, A. & Azouri, L. (1973). Factors associated with broken appointments in an experimental family health center. *Tropical Doctor, 3*, 128-133.

Harris, M. B. & Bruner, C. G. (1971). A comparison of a self-control and a contract procedure for weight control. *Behavior Research, 9*, 347-354.

Hay, W., Hay, L. & Nelson, R. O. (1977). The adaptation of covert modeling procedures to the treatment of chronic alcoholism and obsessive-compulsive behavior: Two case reports. *Behavior Therapy, 8*, 70-76.

Haynes, R. B., Sackett, D. L., Gibson, E. S., Taylor, D. W., Hackett, B. C., Roberts, R. S. & Johnson, A. L. (1976). Improvement of medication compliance in uncontrolled hypertension. *The Lancet, 1*, 1265-1268.

Haynes, R. B., Taylor, D. W. & Sackett, D. L. (1979). *Compliance in health care*. Baltimore: Johns Hopkins University Press.

Haynes, S. N. (1978). *Principles of behavioral assessment*. New York: Gardner Press.

Haynes, S. N. & Wilson, C. C. (1979). *Behavioral assessment*. San Francisco: Jossey-Bass.

Israel, A. C. & Saccone, A. J. (1979). Follow-up effects of choice of mediator and target of reinforcement on weight loss. *Behavior Therapy, 10*, 260-265.

Johnston, J. & Pennypacker, H. S. (1980). *Strategies and tactics of human behavioral research*. Hillsdale, NJ: Erlbaum.

Kanfer, F. H. & Grimm, L. G. (1978). Freedom of choice and behavioral change. *Journal of Consulting and Clinical Psychology, 46*, 873-876.

Kanfer, F. H., Karoly, P. & Newman, A. (1974). Source of feedback, observational learning, and attitude change. *Journal of Personality and Social Psychology, 29*, 30-38.

Kanfer, F. H. & Phillips, J. S. (1969). *Learning foundations of behavior therapy*. New York: John Wiley.

Kazdin, A. E. (1973). Covert modeling and the reduction of avoidance behavior. *Journal of Abnormal Psychology, 81*, 87-95.

Kazdin, A. E. (1974). Comparative effects of some variations of covert modeling. *Journal of Behavior Therapy and Experimental Psychiatry, 5*, 225-231. (a)

Kazdin, A. E. (1974). Covert modeling, model similarity and reduction of avoidance behavior. *Behavior Therapy, 5*, 325-340. (b)

Kazdin, A. E. (1974). The effect of model identify and fear-relevant similarity on covert modeling. *Behavior Therapy, 5*, 624-635. (c)

Kazdin, A. E. (1974). Effects of covert modeling and model reinforcement on assertive behavior. *Journal of Abnormal Psychology, 83*, 240-252. (d)

Kazdin, A. E. (1975). Covert modeling, imagery assessment and assertive behavior. *Journal of Consulting and Clinical Psychology, 43*, 716-724.

Kazdin, A. E. (1976). Assessment of imagery during covert modeling of assertive behavior. *Journal of Behavior Therapy and Experimental Psychiatry, 7*, 213-219. (a)

Kazdin, A. E. (1976). Effects of covert modeling, multiple models, and model reinforcement on assertive behavior. *Behavior Therapy, 7*, 211-222. (b)

Keefe, F. J., Kopel, S. A. & Gordon, S. B. (1978). *A practical guide to behavioral assessment*. New York: Springer.

Kidd, A. H. & Euphrat, J. L. (1971). Why prospective outpatients fail to make or keep appointments. *Journal of Clinical Psychology, 27*, 394-395.

Kingsley, R. G. & Shapiro, J. A. (1977). A comparison of three behavioral programs for the control of obesity in children. *Behavior Therapy, 8*, 30-36.

Krause, M. S. (1966). Comparative effects on continuance of four experimental intake procedures. *Social Casework, 47*, 515-519.

Leitenberg, H. (1975). Feedback and therapist praise during treatment of phobia. *Journal of Consulting and Clinical Psychology, 43*, 396-404.

Leon, G. R. (1976). Current dimensions in the treatment of obesity. *Psychological Bulletin, 83*, 557-578.

Lepper, M. R. (1973). Dissonance, self-perception and honesty in children. *Journal of Personality and Social Psychology, 25*, 65-74.

Levy, R. L. (1977). Relationship of an overt commitment to task compliance in behavior therapy. *Journal of Behavior Therapy and Experimental Psychiatry, 8*, 25-29.

Levy, R. L. (1978). Facilitating patient compliance with medical regimens: An area for social work research and intervention. In N. Bracht (Ed.), *Social work in health care: A guide to professional practice*. New York: The Haworth Press.

Levy, R. L. (1980). The role of social support in patient compliance: A selective review. In R. B. Haynes, M. E. Mattson & T. O. Engebretson, *Patient compliance to prescribed antihypertensive regimens*. NIH Publication No. 81-2102.

Levy, R. L. (1983). Social support and compliance: A selective review and critique of treatment integrity and outcome measurement. *Social Science and Medicine, 17*, 1329-1335.

Levy, R. L. (1985). Social support and compliance: Update. *Journal of Hypertension, 3*, suppl. 1, 45-49.

Levy, R. L. (in press). Social support and compliance: Salient methodological problems in compliance research. *Compliance in health care*.

Levy, R. L. & Carter, R. D. (1976). Compliance with practitioner instigations. *Social Work, 21*, 188-193.

Levy, R. L. & Claravell, V. (1977). Differential effects of a phone reminder on patients with long and short between-visit intervals. *Medical Care, 15*, 435-438.

Levy, R. L. & Clark, H. (1980). The use of an overt commitment to enhance compliance. A cautionary note. *Journal of Behavior Therapy and Experimental Psychiatry, 11*, 105-107.

Levy, R. L., Yamashita, D. & Pow, G. (1979). Relationship of an overt commitment to the frequency and speed of compliance with symptom reporting. *Medical Care, 17*.

Lewis, S. (1974). A comparison of behavior therapy techniques in the reduction of fearful avoidance behavior. *Behavior Therapy, 5*, 648-655.

Liebert, R. M., Hanratty, M. & Hill, J. H. (1969). Effects of role structure and training method on the adoption of a self-imposed standard. *Child Development, 40*, 93-101.

Locke, E. A., Cartledge, H. & Koeppel, J. (1968). Motivational effects of knowledge of results: A goal-setting phenomenon. *Psychological Bulletin, 70*, 478-485.

Lovitt, T. C. & Curtiss, K. (1969). Academic response rate as a function of teacher- and self-imposed contingencies. *Journal of Applied Behavior Analysis, 2*, 49-53.

Lowe, K. & Lutzker, J. R. (1979). Increasing compliance to a medical regimen with a juvenile diabetic. *Behavior Therapy, 10*, 57-64.

Mahoney, M. J., Moura, N. G. & Wade, T. C. (1973). Relative efficacy of self-reward, self-punishment, and self-monitoring techniques for weight loss. *Journal of Consulting and Clinical Psychology, 40*, 404-407.

Maiman, L. A. & Becker, M. H. (1974). The health belief model: Origins and correlates in psychological theory. *Health Education Monographs, 2*, 255-469.

Mann, R. A. (1972). The behavior-therapeutic use of contingency contracting to control an adult behavior problem: Weight control. *Journal of Applied Behavior Analysis, 5*, 99-109.

McFall, R. M. & Marston, A. R. (1970). An experimental investigation of behavior rehearsal in assertive training. *Journal of Abnormal Psychology, 76*, 295-303.

McKenney, J. M., Slining, J. M., Henderson, H. R., Devins, D. & Barr, M. (1973). The effect of clinical pharmacy services on patients with essential hypertension. *Circulation, 48*, 1104-1111.

Miller, W. R. (1978). Behavioral treatment of problem drinkers: A comparative outcome study of three controlled drinking therapies. *Journal of Consulting and Clinical Psychology, 46*, 74-86.

Moulding, T. (1961). Preliminary study of the pill calendar as a method of improving self-administration of drugs. *American Review of Respiratory Disease, 84*, 284-287.

Nazarian, L. F., Machuber, J., Charney, E. & Coulter, M. D. (1974). Effect of a mailed appointment reminder on appointment keeping. *Pediatrics, 53*, 349-351.

Nesse, M. & Nelson, R. O. (1977). Variations of covert modeling on cigarette smoking. *Cognitive Therapy and Research, 1*, 343-354.

Olson, D. G. & Levy, R. L. (1981). Enhancing high risk children's utilization of dental services. *American Journal of Public Health, 71*, 631-634.

Peterson, L. Homer, A. L. & Wonderlich, S. (1982). The integrity of independent variables in behavior analysis. *Journal of Applied Behavior Analysis, 15*, 477-492.

Phillips, R. (1966). Self-administered systematic desensitization. *Journal of Consulting and Clinical Psychology, 18*, 491-501.

Rappaport, J., Gross, T. & Lepper, C. (1973). Modeling, sensitivity training and instruction. *Journal of Consulting and Clinical Psychology, 40*, 99-107.

Rosenstock, I. M. (1966). Why people use health services. *Milbank Memorial Fund Quarterly, 44*, 94-124.

Saccone, A. J. & Israel, A. C. (1978). Effects of experimenter versus significant other-controlled reinforcement and choice of target behaviors on weight loss. *Behavior Therapy, 9*, 271-278.

Sackett, D. L., Haynes, R. B., Gibson, E. S., Hackett, B. C., Taylor, D. W., Roberts, R. S. & Johnson, A. L. (1975). Randomized clinical trial of strategies for improving medication compliance in primary hypertensive. *The Lancet, 1*, 1205-1207.

Schulman, B. (1979). Active patient orientation and outcomes in hypertensive treatment. *Medical Care, 17*, 267-280.

Shelton, J. L. & Levy, R. L. (1979). Home practice activities and compliance: Two sources of error variance in behavioral research. *Journal of Applied Behavior Analysis, 12*, 324.

Shelton, J. & Levy, R. L. (1981). *Behavioral assignments and treatment compliance: A handbook of clinical strategies.* Champaign, IL: Research Press(a).

Shelton, J. L. & Levy, R. L. (1981). A survey of the reported use of assigned homework activities in contemporary behavior therapy. *The Behavior Therapist, 4*, 12-14(b).

Shepard, D. S. & Moseley, T. A. (1976). Mailed vs. telephoned appointment reminders to reduce broken appointments in a hospital outpatient department. *Medical Care, 14*, 268-273.

Steckel, S. B. & Swain, M. A. (1977). Contracting with patients to improve compliance. *Hospitals, 51*(23), 81-84.

Stokols, D. (1975). The reduction of cardiovascular risk: An application of social learning perspectives. In A. J. Enelow & J. B. Henderson (Eds.), *Applying behavioral science to cardiovascular risk.* Dallas: American Heart Association.

Stuart, R. B. & Davis, B. (1972). *Slim chance in a fat world.* Champaign, IL: Research Press.

Suinn, R. M. (1977). Behavioral methods at the Winter Olympic Games. *Behavior Therapy, 8*, 283-284.

Svarstad, B. (1976). Physician-patient communication and patient conformity with medical advice. In D. Mechanic (Ed.), *The growth of bureaucratic medicine.* New York: John Wiley & Sons.

Takala, J., Niemela, N., Rosti, J. & Silvers, K. (1979). Improving compliance with therapeutic regimens in hypertensive patients in a community health center. *Circulation, 59*, 540-543.

Wilson, G. T. & Evans, I. M. (1972). The therapist-client relationship in behavior therapy. In A. S. Gurman & A. M. Razin (Eds.), *The therapist's contribution to effective psychotherapy: An empirical approach.* Elmsford, NY: Pergamon Press.

Wurtele, S. K., Galanos, A. N. & Roberts, M. C. (1978). Self-directed treatment for premature ejaculation. *Journal of Consulting and Clinical Psychology, 46*, 1234-1241.

Zitter, R. E. & Freemouw, W. J. (1978). Individual vs. partner consequation for weight loss. *Behavior Therapy, 9*, 808-813.

Clinical Research
in Sexual Dysfunctions:
Social Work Contributions

Dianne F. Harrison

SUMMARY. This article reviews the extent to which social workers have contributed to the empirical evaluation of behavioral therapy in the treatment of psychosexual dysfunctions. To better evaluate the social work contributions, an overview of the status of research and findings in the field of sex therapy is discussed, including recent questions which have been raised regarding effectiveness. Only three controlled outcome studies were located which had at least one social work author. These studies are examined in terms of congruency with previous reports and overall quality of the contribution to knowledge development in behavioral sex therapy. Additional social work contributions in a variety of "non-traditional" sexual problem areas are briefly highlighted.

Social workers across a variety of practice settings frequently encounter sex-related problems of clients and are increasingly providing sex education and/or sex therapy services. To what extent have they contributed to the research literature in this area? The purpose of this article is to address this question by reviewing contributions made by social workers to the empirical evaluation of behavioral treatments of sexual dysfunctions. While work done by social workers in other sexual problem areas will be briefly highlighted, the current focus is primarily on the outcome of behavioral treatment for the "psychosexual dysfunc-

Dianne F. Harrison, Associate Professor, School of Social Work, Florida State University, Tallahassee, Florida 32306.

tions" or "inhibitions in sexual desire or the psychophysiological changes that characterize the sexual response cycle" (American Psychiatric Association, 1980, p. 261). The rationale for this limitation in scope is two-fold: first, due to the alleged prevalence of these types of sexual problems among couples seeking marital therapy (Stuart & Hammond, 1980) and among the general population (Masters & Johnson, 1970; Frank et al., 1978); and second, the fact that several investigations have questioned the effectiveness of sex therapy in general (Kilmann & Mills, 1983; Zilbergeld & Kilmann, 1984) and of behavioral sex therapy techniques in particular (Marks, 1981; Friedman & Hogan, 1985). In order to provide a context within which the social work contributions can be better evaluated, an overview of the current status of research and issues in the field of sex therapy and behavioral sex therapy will also be given.

SOCIAL WORK IN OTHER SEXUAL PROBLEM AREAS

Since the early 1970s there has been an enormous proliferation of human sexuality literature by social workers which has covered a broad spectrum of topics. These topics have included such areas as sexual oppression (Gochros, 1972; Gochros & Gochros, 1977; Gochros, Gochros & Fischer, 1986); sexual abuse (Conte, 1982; Chandler, 1982; Jehu, Gazan & Klassen, 1985); homosexuality (Berger, 1977; 1983; Duehn & Mayadas, 1977); physical disabilities (Harrison, 1979; Askwith, 1983); aging (Wasow & Loeb, 1975; Marson, 1983); self-help (Gochros & Fischer, 1980); and sex education for social workers (Abramowitz, 1971; Gochros & Schultz, 1972; Chilman, 1975; Kunkel, 1979; Schlesingers, 1983). With the exception of the Duehn and Mayadas article (1977), this literature has been non-data based, clinically oriented and descriptive in nature. As a result, while social workers have made what may be significant contributions to the clinical and educational literature in a variety of "non-traditional" sexual problems areas, the empirical evidence is sparse. Although the profession is not unique in this deficit (see, for example, Hogan, 1978; and Marks, 1981), it is clear that the need exists for well-designed outcome studies in these areas.

Current Status of Sex Therapy and Behavioral Sex Therapy with Psychosexual Dysfunctions

Before examining the role played by social workers in the evaluation of behavioral treatments of sexual dysfunction, the current status of clinical research on effectiveness of sex therapy will be described. The term sex therapy has been used to refer to "relatively brief, directive, symptom-oriented approaches" (Zilbergeld & Kilmann, 1984, p. 319) with behavioral sex therapy referring to "a direct approach to the modification of sexual behavior . . . (with) an emphasis on the empirical validation of treatment techniques" (Friedman & Hogan, 1985, p. 418). Because both terms have implied non-psychodynamic approaches, and so-called behavioral treatments frequently have included techniques which are quasi-behavioral and not based on behavioral principles or laboratory experiments, the terms sex therapy and behavioral sex therapy have become relatively indistinguishable. Further, critical issues in the research literature which will be reviewed apply equally to the general field of sex therapy and to the specific area of behavioral treatments for sexual dysfunctions. Where differences exist, they will be noted.

The field of sex therapy has been described as "still in a pre-scientific state," directed largely by "clinical wisdom" and the art of practice (Stuart & Hammond, 1980). The enthusiasm of the 1970s and advocacy of behavioral sex therapy prompted by earlier dramatic success rates have waned considerably in the 1980s. Although behavioral approaches remain the treatment of choice based on the evidence (Barlow, 1985), the previous high success rates have not been replicated and significant relapse rates at long term follow-up have been reported (Heiman & LoPiccolo, 1983; DeAmicis, Goldberg, LoPiccolo, Friedman & Davies, 1984). Another factor accounting for treatment failures and for the lessened enthusiasm for behavioral approaches has to do with the apparent shift in problems presented to therapists; i.e., from the "pure" dysfunctions (orgasmic, erectile, or ejaculatory problems) to the more complex, sometimes multiple, dysfunctions often accompanied by severe individual and relationship difficulties (Friedman & Hogan, 1985). For example, there has been an increase in the incidence of low sex desire, both as a single presenting problem and in combination with other problems (LoPiccolo, 1980; Hawton, 1982), the prognosis of which is poorer than for the excitement and orgasmic dysfunctions (Friedman & Hogan, 1985).

EFFECTIVENESS OF SEX THERAPY

The incidence of complex, multiple dysfunctions notwithstanding, the research literature in sex therapy has been characterized as "primitive" (Hogan, 1978) and "shakey" (Heiman & LoPiccolo, 1983), consisting largely of uncontrolled case studies (Zilbergeld & Kilmann, 1984). However, while the clinical management of sexual dysfunctions has forged ahead of the evidence, several reviewers have tentatively summarized what is currently known and unknown with respect to effectiveness based on the case reports and controlled studies which do exist (Hogan, 1978; Marks, 1981; and Zilbergeld & Kilmann, 1984). These findings have to do with treatment format, interventive techniques, client characteristics, success and failure rates with various target problems, and spillover effects.

Format. Both the Marks (1981) and Zilbergeld and Kilmann (1984) reviews reported that there was no evidence to support the use of two rather than one therapist in sex treatment, a finding which contraindicates the rather expensive use of dual sex therapists. Further, neither an individual or couple or group treatment approach has been found superior. While results from some group treatment experiments have been positive (Marks, 1981) and probably more efficient and more cost effective, disadvantages related to confidentiality, privacy, and group coercion in the group treatment of sexual dysfunctions also have to be considered (Barbach, 1979). With respect to frequency of sessions, outcomes have been similar with both spaced (usually weekly) and daily sessions (Heiman & Lopiccolo, 1983). Finally, insufficient data exist to draw conclusions about the use of surrogate partners (Zilbergeld & Kilmann, 1984).

Techniques. In his review of eighteen controlled studies, Marks reported that a "behavioral Masters and Johnson" approach was superior to other methods (1981, p. 750). Central components of the behavioral approach typically entail anxiety reduction techniques and sexual skills training. Marks concluded that desensitization in fantasy produced weak effects and directed sexual skills training was "probably more potent than contrasting procedures" (1981, p. 754). Similarly, the Zilbergeld and Kilmann (1984) review concluded that, in general, direct work on a sexual problem (completing tasks or corrective exercises to effect change) was more effective than simply talking about or dealing with the presumed causes of a problem. Other than the stop-start or squeeze methods for premature ejaculation, anxiety reduction techniques for erectile dysfunctions, and anxiety reduction and stimulation by self or partner for female orgasmic dysfunctions, additional knowledge about the effects of particular types of direct work is lacking. Which particular types of anxiety reduction techniques are more effective in general or with specific clients, for example, is unknown. Likewise, the effects of such techniques as intercourse bans, Kegel exercises, sensate-focus, and assertiveness and communication training are unknown (Zilbergeld & Kilmann, 1984).

Client characteristics. Several client characteristics have been found to be associated with either the success or failure of sex therapy. A history of psychiatric treatment and the presence of severe marital difficulties, for example, have been related to a high dropout rate (Marks, 1981). In another review, Jehu suggested that severe discord between partners was probably "the most notable contraindication" for sex therapy (1980, p. 23), most likely due to noncompliance with treatment assignments. Based on a "consensus among therapists" rather than controlled research, Zilbergeld and Kilmann also suggested that clients who actively participated in treatment and were compliant with homework assignments are more likely to achieve the best results (1984, p. 322). As will be discussed further later, a client's presenting problem is a critical determinant of treatment outcome, with certain target problems having a much greater likelihood of success than others (Jehu, 1980; Marks, 1981; Zilbergeld & Kilmann, 1984).

Target problems. Behavioral sex therapy has been found to be most successful (70-100%) in the treatment of females with primary orgasmic dysfunction (Zilbergeld & Kilmann, 1984). Orgasm has been typically achieved through masturbation following 8-15 sessions, with the majority of women eventually capable of orgasm with partner stimulation. Treatment of premature ejaculation has also been successful (50-100%), meaning that males in sexual interactions with partners have increased their ability to delay orgasm (Zilbergeld & Kilmann, 1984). Results in the treatment of erectile failure and secondary or situational anorgasmia have been less successful, ranging from 0-75%. Data are insufficient to justify conclusions about effectiveness in the problems of ejaculatory inhibition, dyspareunia, and low sex desire (Zilbergeld & Kilmann, 1984). With the exception of primary anorgasmia, relapse rates for the remaining target problems have ranged from 0-50% at long-term follow-up (Zilbergeld & Kilmann, 1984; Friedman & Hogan, 1985). Finally, even in successful cases, improvement has generally been incomplete in that changes produced have not resulted in a complete "cure" or resolution of the problem (Marks, 1981; Zilbergeld & Kilmann, 1984).

"Spillover" effects. Even in cases where target sexual problems have not shown significant improvement, side effects in other areas have been found. Improved changes have occurred in such areas as sexual satisfaction, communication, marital adjustment, and sexual anxiety (Zilbergeld & Kilmann, 1984). However, in a thus far unreplicated exploratory study, Payn and Wakefield (1982) found negative effects on the marital relationship for some couples following the female's treatment of primary anorgasmia; these effects were attributed to the lack of partner involvement in treatment.

Methodological Issues

Even in controlled research studies, methodological problems seem to be pervasive in the sex therapy literature. One major difficulty is the lack of a standard nomenclature, evident in the wide range of definitions and descriptions of sexual dysfunctions used (Hogan, 1978; Stuart & Hammond, 1980). As a result, comparability across studies is problematic. Similarly, the criteria used to evaluate success or failure (for example, patient reports versus partner reports versus behavioral indices, or global categories versus specific referents) have been inconsistent (Hogan, 1978; Pervin & Leiblum, 1980). The effects of a number of client variables, such as specific type and length of marital or psychological problems present, partner availability, selection criteria, and problem onset, have not been identified (Hogan, 1978; Hawton, 1982). Follow-ups have been incomplete or contaminated (Marks, 1981) and the question of generalizability (for example, orgasm with masturbation or during intercourse) is not typically addressed (Pervin & Leiblum, 1980). Another weakness in the research literature is the existence of only a few controlled component analyses such that it remains virtually unknown exactly which elements of a treatment package are most effective with different problems (Hogan, 1978; Stuart & Hammond, 1980). A related problem is the inadequacy of descriptions given of treatment techniques. Studies which were reportedly evaluating one technique, have included other techniques in a package without examining their effect on outcome (Stuart & Hammond, 1980).

As a result, the field of sex therapy is in need of controlled clinical outcome studies which address these problems. Hogan (1978) has recommended the use of factorial designs which examine and control for client variables, treatment components and mode of therapy. As mentioned earlier, data are also needed on the effects of treatment compliance and long-term maintenance, particularly given the incidence of relapse. Finally, systematic replications of single-case designs can produce information about outcome effectiveness in behavioral sex therapy in an efficient and clinically feasible manner yet have been relatively unexploited in this area.

SOCIAL WORK CONTRIBUTIONS

To examine the extent to which social workers have contributed to the research in behavioral sex therapy, a computer-assisted literature review was conducted for the years 1970-1985. To be included in this analysis, studies had to: (1) report on the outcome of behavioral sex therapy with one or more of the psychosexual dysfunctions; (2) have some type of control feature in the research design; and (3) have at least one social work author (as indicated by academic degree). While seven studies were located which met the first and last criteria, control features existed in only three of the seven. The controlled studies will be examined in the next section with respect to degree of congruency with previous reports and the overall quality of the contribution to knowledge development in behavioral sex therapy.

Controlled Studies

Table 1 summarizes the outcome studies which met all three criteria described earlier. Interestingly, none of these studies were done in the United States. Two of the three (Brender, Libman, Burstein & Takefman, 1983; Libman, Fichter, Brender, Burstein, Cohen & Binik, 1984) were conducted in the same setting: the Sexual Dysfunction Service in the Department of Psychiatry, Jewish General Hospital, Montreal. The social work contributor in these two studies (Burstein) was third and fourth author, respectively. The third study (Adkins & Jehu, 1985) was carried out at a sexual dysfunction clinic in Manitoba, Canada. In two (Brender et al., 1983; Adkins & Jehu, 1985) treatment was administered either in full or in part by an MSW. Although Adkins and Jehu described the therapist as "a clinical psychology student (E.A.)" (1985, p. 120), Adkins is also an ACSW. Therapists in the Libman et al. (1984) article were described only as: "experienced sex therapists" and by gender. All three studies examined the spillover effects of treatment on non-targeted individual and relationship functioning.

In a clinical investigation of behavioral sex therapy outcome, Brender et al. (1983) reported "substantial improvements in the presenting complaint" at follow-up (p. 351). This quasi-experimental study incorporated a pre-post with comparison group design, and used multiple self-report outcome measures which were administered two times during both pre- and post therapy and once at follow-up. Unfortunately, serious methodological flaws hinder confident interpretation and generalizability of results. These weaknesses include a failure to specify client selection criteria the use of an extremely heterogeneous sample, incomplete follow-up, lack of specificity of the treatment pack-

Table 1

Controlled Studies by Social Work Authors

Study	Treatment Target	# of Subjects	# of Treatment Sessions	Length of Follow-up	Outcome	Comments
Brender, Libman, Burstein, & Takefman (1983)	Range of targets included	38 couples	Varied by individual case	8 mos.	Positive change on 6 of 12 sexual behavior items, 3 of which did not maintain at follow-up; increased global sexual happiness for treated group; improvement in target problem ranged from 25-100%; differences between clinical and non-problem group on sexual items at pre and post.	21 couples received treatment, compared with 17 well-adjusted couples matched on demographics; 11 couples completed follow-up.
Libman, Fichten, Brender, Burstein, Cohen, & Binik (1984)	Secondary orgasmic dysfunction	23 couples	15	3 mos.	For all 3 treatment conditions: positive effects on global sexual satisfaction and sexual behavior measures; improvements in sexual behavior inconsistently maintained at follow-up. Largest gain in noncoital sexual activities; increases in rate of orgasm not maintained at follow-up. Few differences between therapy conditions; standard couples therapy generally favored. No effects on marital satisfaction or personality variables.	Compared 3 therapy formats (couple vs group vs minimal contact bibliotherapy) using cognitive behavioral sex therapy; incomplete follow-up.
Adkins & Jehu (1985)	Primary Anorgasmia	6 couples	10	1 and 6 mos.	3 out of 6 women achieved orgasm during treatment and maintained at follow-up; improvement in non-targeted behavior observed for all S's.	Non-concurrent multiple baseline across-subjects design used; repeated measures taken after each treatment phase.

Note. + indicates known social work author.

113

age and use of multiple treatment packages, and in the authors' own admission, the use of questionable and less than rigorous data analytic procedures. As a result, the study findings must be interpreted so cautiously that they add little to the state of knowledge in the field.

In a much improved study apparently conducted by the same research team, Libman et al. (1984) used a factorial design to compare three therapeutic formats each using a structured cognitive-behavioral sex therapy program to treat secondary orgasmic dysfunction. As noted in Table 1, favorable effects at post-test were found for all three treatment conditions; infrequent and small differences were found between conditions with standard couple therapy generally favored. Success rates for females achieving orgasm during a variety of sexual activities ranged from a high of 66% (during masturbation) to a low of 6% (intercourse, female on top). These rates are congruent with those cited in earlier reviews (0-75%; Zilbergeld & Kilmann, 1984). Multiple outcome criteria were employed by Libman et al. including both subjective satisfaction and behavioral measures. The authors clearly defined client selection criteria, target problem, and treatment conditions. They also discussed the implications for cost effectiveness of the different therapy formats. Unspecified, however, were exactly how couples were assigned to treatment conditions and therapist characteristics (other than "experience" and gender). Follow-up was of relatively short duration (3 months) and was incomplete to the point that treatment effects could not be evaluated in some ANOVA comparisons, a serious shortcoming given relapse rates described earlier. Finally, insufficient data were presented in the article to allow the reader to critically evaluate the findings (for example, results from ANOVA comparisons are displayed only in terms of means and probability levels). Overall, this study satisfies many of the earlier methodological complaints seen in the literature and provides important replication data regarding the relative efficacy of behavioral treatment and the merits of couple vs group vs minimal contact therapy formats. Except for the issue of maintenance of treatment gains, the authors appear to have fulfilled their research intent in a methodologically sound manner, with improvements needed mainly in the areas of clarity and thoroughness in presenting results.

The Adkins and Jehu (1985) study represents one of the few attempts in the field to conduct a component analysis of a behavioral treatment package for the problem of primary anorgasmia. The need for this type of research in sex therapy was discussed earlier and is particularly relevant to the problem of primary orgasmic dysfunction in light of the high treatment success rates (70-100%) and almost nonexistent relapse rates (Zilbergeld & Kilmann, 1984). In a methodologically sound design using multiple outcome measures, the authors demonstrated the effectiveness of the use of a vibrator in the "Partner-Involvement with no Intercourse" phase of treatment in helping women achieve orgasm (p. 119). Screening procedures and treatment phases were clearly described. Unfortunately, only three of the six women were able to attain orgasm during the program, a success rate (50%) somewhat lower than those previously cited. The low success rate was attributed by the authors to various characteristics of the subject pool, failure to complete homework assignments, therapist effects, problems in initial diagnosis, and/or the use of a highly structured (non-individualized) course of treatment. Data from the study were reported incompletely; results related to frequency of orgasm were presented graphically with the remaining data presented only in terms of percentages and number of subjects reporting increases, decreases, or no change on outcome measures. Overall, this study is a useful contribution to the literature in that at least some initial information was provided regarding the relative contributions of various treatment components as well as further information about treatment effects on nontarget areas. The study left unanswered, however, numerous questions about essential versus incidental treatment components, and ordering or sequence of treatment effects.

To summarize, two of the three studies reviewed appear to make valuable contributions to the research literature in the behavioral treatment of sexual dysfunction. Four additional outcome studies which were located and authored by at least one social worker (Waggoner, Mudd & Shearer, 1978; Barback &

Flaherty, 1980; Kaplan, Fyer & Novick, 1982; Payn & Wakefield, 1982) were excluded for lack of control features in the research design. It should be noted that the criteria for inclusion also eliminated three texts, authored by social workers (Fischer & Gochros, 1977a, 1977b; Jehu, 1979, Stuart, 1980), that present behavioral approaches to the treatment of sexual (and in the case of Stuart, marital) dysfunction which have some degree of empirical validation. The criteria also eliminated two assessment devices which were devised and tested by social workers (Stuart, Stuart, Maurice & Szasz, 1975; Hudson, Harrison & Crosscup, 1981) and used in several outcome studies as well as Gochros and Fischer's (1980) behaviorally-based sexual enhancement self-help book.

CONCLUSION

Contrary to Szasz's (1980) assertion that the "so-called sexual dysfunctions" which are psychogenic in nature, are not medical diseases or problems requiring sex therapy (p. 13), social workers and other mental health professionals have provided and will probably continue to provide a number of interventions aimed at alleviating such difficulties.

This article addressed the question, "To what extent have social workers contributed to the research literature in the area of behavioral sex therapy?" On the basis of the current review the response is discouraging. Only three controlled outcome studies were located in this area, two of which were judged as valuable. In only one study was the senior author a social worker. Relative to the number of controlled studies conducted by social workers evaluating practice in all areas as reported by Fischer (N = 11; 1973), Wood (N = 22; 1978), Reid and Hanrahan (N = 22; 1982), and Rubin (N = 12; 1985), the small number in the area of behavioral sex therapy is not surprising. This is not to discount the fact, however, that there continues to be a tremendous need for additional research in this area. Given the profession's demands for demonstrations of practice effectiveness and the current status of knowledge about sex therapy, social work researchers have not only the opportunity, but also the obligation to make significant contributions to the treatment of sexual problems.

REFERENCES

Abramowitz, N. W. (1971). Human sexuality in the social work curriculum. *The Family Coordinator, 20*, 349-354.

Adkins, E. & Jehu, D. (1985). Analysis of a treatment program for primary orgastic dysfunction. *Behavior Research and Therapy, 23*, 119-126.

American Psychiatric Association (1980). *Diagnostic and Statistical Manual of Mental Disorders* (DSM III). 3rd ed.; Washington, DC: Author.

Askwith, J. (1983). The role of social work in enhancing the sexuality of the physically handicapped. *Journal of Social Work and Human Sexuality, 1*, 83-93.

Barbach, L. (1979). Ethical issues in group treatment of sexual dysfunctions. *Journal of Sex Education and Therapy, 1*, 65-67.

Barbach, L. & Flaherty, M. (1980). Group treatment of situationally orgasmic women. *Journal of Sex and Marital Therapy, 6*, 19-29.

Barlow, D. H. (Ed.) (1985). *Clinical handbook of psychological disorders*. New York: The Guilford Press.

Berger, R. M. (1977). An advocate model for intervention with homosexuals. *Social Work, 22*(4), 280-283.

Berger, R. M. (1983). Health care for lesbians and gays: What social workers should know. *Journal of Social Work and Human Sexuality, 1*, 59-73.

Brender, W., Libman, E., Burstein, R. & Takefman, J. (1983). Behavioral sex therapy: a preliminary study of its effectiveness in a clinical setting. *The Journal of Sex Research, 19*, 351-365.

Chandler, S. M. (1982). Knowns and unknowns in sexual abuse of children. *Journal of Social Work & Human Sexuality, 1*, 51-68.

Chilman, C. (1975). Some knowledge bases regarding human sexuality. *Journal of Education for Social Work, 11*, 11-17.

Conte, J. R. (1982). Sexual abuse of children: Enduring issues for social work. *Journal of Social Work & Human Sexuality, 1*, 1-19.

DeAmicis, L. A., Goldberg, D. C., LoPiccolo, J., Friedman, J. M. & Davies, L. (1984). Three-year follow-up of couples evaluated for sexual dysfunction. *Journal of Sex and Marital Therapy, 10*(4), 215-218.

Duehn, W. D. & Mayadas, N. S. (1977). The use of stimulus/modeling videotapes in assertive training for homosexuals. In J. Fischer & H.L. Gochros (Eds.), *Handbook of behavior therapy with sexual problems, Approaches to specific problems*, Vol. II. New York: Pergamon Press.

Fischer, J. (1973). Is casework effective: A review. *Social Work, 18*, 5-20.

Fischer, J. & Gochros, H. L. (1977a). *Handbook of behavior therapy with sexual problems; Vol. I, General procedures*. New York: Pergamon Press.

Fischer, J. & Gochros, H. L. (1977b). *Handbook of behavior therapy with sexual problems; Vol. II, Approaches to specific problems*. New York: Pergamon Press.

Frank, E., Anderson, C. & Rubenstein, D. (1978). Frequency of sexual dysfunction in "normal" couples. *New England Journal of Medicine, 299*, 111-115.

Friedman, J. M. & Hogan, D. R. (1985). Sexual dysfunction & low sexual desire. In D. H. Barlow (Ed.), *Clinical handbook of psychological disorders*, pp. 417-461. New York: The Guilford Press.

Gochros, H. (1972). The sexually oppressed. *Social Work, 17*(2), 16-23.

Gochros, H. L. & Schlutz, L. G. (1972). *Human sexuality and social work*. New York: Association Press.

Gochros, H. & Gochros, J. (Eds.) (1977). *The sexually oppressed*. New York: Association Press.

Gochros, H. L. & Fischer, J. (1980). *Treat yourself to a better sex life*. Englewood Cliffs, NJ: Prentice-Hall.

Gochros, H., Gochros, J. S. & Fischer, J. (Eds.) (1986). *Helping the sexually oppressed*. Englewood Cliffs, NJ: Prentice-Hall.

Harrison, D. F. (1979). Sexuality and the physically handicapped: Some guidelines for social workers. In D. Kunkel (Ed.), *Sexual issues in social work: Emerging concerns in education and practice*. Honolulu, Hawaii: School of Social Work, University of Hawaii.

Hawton, K. (1982). The behavioral treatment of sexual dysfunction. *British Journal of Psychiatry, 140*, 94-101.

Heiman, J. R. & Lopiccolo, J. (1983). Clinical outcome of sex therapy effects of daily versus weekly treatment. *Archives of General Psychiatry, 40*, 443-449.

Hogan, D. R. (1978). The effectiveness of sex therapy: A review of the literature. In J. Lopiccolo & L. Lopiccolo (Eds.), *Handbook of sex therapy*. New York: Plenum Press.

Hudson, W. W., Harrison, D. F. & Crosscup, P. (1981). A short-form scale to measure sexual discord in dyadic relationships. *Journal of Sex Research, 17*, 157-174.

Jehu, D. (1979). *Sexual dysfunctions: A behavioral approach to causation, assessment and treatment*. New York: Wiley.

Jehu, D. (1980). Recent developments in therapy for sexual dysfunction. *Australian Psychologist, 15*, 19-31.

Jehu, D., Gazan, M. & Klassen, C. (1985). Common therapeutic targets among women who were sexually abused in childhood. *Journal of Social Work & Human Sexuality, 4*, 25-45.

Kaplan, H. S., Fyer, A. J. & Novick, A. (1983). The treatment of sexual phobias: The combined use of antipanic medication and sex therapy. *Journal of Sex & Marital Therapy, 8*, 3-28.

Kilmann, P. R. & Mills, K. H. (1983). *All about sex therapy*. New York: Plenum.

Kunkel, D. (Ed.) (1979). *Sexual issues in social work: Emerging concerns in education and practice*. Honolulu, Hawaii: School of Social Work, University of Hawaii.

Libman, E., Fichten, C. S., Brender, W., Burstein, R., Cohen, J. & Binik, Y. M. (1984). A comparison of three therapeutic formats in the treatment of secondary orgasmic dysfunction. *Journal of Sex and Marital Therapy, 10*, 147-159.

LoPiccolo, L. (1980). Low sexual desire. In S. R. Leiblum & L. A. Pervin (Eds.), *Handbook of sex therapy*, pp. 187-194. New York: Plenum.

Marks, I. (1981). Review of behavioral psychotherapy, II: Sexual disorders. *American Journal of Psychiatry, 138*(6, June), 750-756.

Marson, S. M. (1983). Sexuality among the aging: Problems and solutions. *Journal of Social Work and Human Sexuality, 1*, 95-109.

Masters, W. H. & Johnson, V. D. (1970). *Human sexual inadequacy*. Boston: Little, Brown and Co.

Payn, N. & Wakefield, J. (1982). The effect of group treatment of primary orgasmic dysfunction on the marital relationship. *Journal of Sex and Marital Therapy, 8*, 135-150.

Pervin, L. A. & Leiblum, S. R. (1980). Conclusion: Overview of some critical issues in the evaluation and treatment of sexual dysfunctions. In S. R. Leiblum & L. A. Pervin (Eds.), *Principles and practice of sex therapy*. New York: Guilford Press.

Reid, W. J. & Hanrahan, P. (1982). Recent evaluation of social work: Grounds for optimism. *Social Work, 27*, 328-340.

Rubin, A. (1985). Practice effectiveness: More grounds for optimism. *Social Work, 30*, 469-476.

Schlesinger, B. (1983). Teaching human sexuality to graduate social work students: A decade review 1971-1982. *Journal of Social Work and Human Sexuality, 1,* 7-16.

Stuart, F., Stuart, R. B., Maurice, W. L. & Szasz, G. (1975). *Sexual adjustment inventory.* Champaign, IL: Research Press.

Stuart, F. M. & Hammond, D. C. (1980). Sex therapy. In R. B. Stuart, *Helping couples change, A social learning approach to marital therapy.* New York: Guilford Press.

Stuart, R. B. (1980). *Helping couples change, A social learning approach to marital therapy.* New York: Guilford Press.

Szasz, T. (1980). *Sex by prescription.* New York: Doubleday.

Waggoner, R. W., Mudd, E. H. & Shearer, M. L. (1978). Training dual sex teams for rapid treatment of sexual dysfunction: A pilot program. In J. LoPiccolo & L. LoPiccolo (Eds.), *Handbook of sex therapy,* pp. 499-509. New York: Plenum.

Wasow, M. & Loeb, M. B. (1975). Sexuality in nursing homes. In I. Burnside (Ed.), *Sexuality and aging.* Los Angeles: University of Southern California Press.

Wood, K. M. (1978). Casework effectiveness: A new look at the research evidence. *Social Work, 23,* 437-458.

Zilbergeld, B. & Kilmann, P. R. (1984). The scope and effectiveness of sex therapy. *Psychotherapy, 21,* 319-326.

Evaluating a Social Learning Approach to Teaching Adolescents About Alcohol and Driving: A Multiple Variable Evaluation

John S. Wodarski

SUMMARY. The variables influencing adolescent drinking and its consequences are reviewed. A unique educational technique, "Teams-Games-Tournaments," is described in relation to its utility for teaching adolescents about alcohol use and misuse. The implementation and components of the evaluation of the comprehensive program are detailed.

Alcohol studies are not a new area of research. However, within the broad area of alcohol-related literature, there are relatively few reports of studies directed at alcohol abuse by adolescents. Moreover, the majority of data reported are descriptive rather than analytic, and a large percentage is conflictual and ambiguous. Ironically, it is during the adolescent years that the issue of the role alcohol will play in one's life is initially confronted. There is a crucial need therefore for teenagers to have a broad foundation of accurate knowledge to draw upon when

John S. Wodarski, PhD, Director, Research Center, School of Social Work, University of Georgia, Athens, Georgia 30602.

Portions of this paper were presented at the annual meeting of the American Psychological Association, Division 38, Toronto, Canada, August 1984.

Preparation of this manuscript was facilitated by a grant from the United States Department of Transportation (National Highway Traffic Safety Administration contract number DTRS5683-C-00053), the University of Georgia School of Social Work and the University of Georgia Research Foundation, Inc.

making the decisions of when and if to begin drinking, how much to drink, how often, with whom, and where. How best to approach adolescents about the subject of drinking remains to be determined.

To no one's surprise in our increasingly fast-paced world, adolescents are coming into contact with alcohol at earlier ages, and the use of alcohol has increased. According to the 1981 U.S. Department of Health and Human Services Report to the Congress on Alcohol and Health, a 1978 national survey of youths revealed that 87% of tenth through twelfth grade students had consumed alcohol (U.S. Department of Health and Human Services, 1981). It was also found that drinking increased substantially from ages 15 to 17, and that a substantial number of youths were heavy drinkers by age 15. Of the adolescents surveyed, 15% drank once per week (consuming five drinks or more), 31% experienced drunkenness six times or more per year, and 2% reported adverse consequences as a result of drinking excessively two times or more per year. Perhaps most alarming of all is that a startling 31.2% of those surveyed were classified as alcohol misusers (defined as consuming five drinks or more three times per week or more). It can be concluded from this report that youths *are* making decisions concerning the use of alcohol, and that many are finding themselves in a spiraling cycle of increased drinking that occasionally results in negative consequences.

Other recent studies support these findings and point out that alcohol is the most widely used drug among American youths (Abelson, 1977; Johnson, 1977; Rachal, Maisto, Guess & Hubbard, 1982). For example, in the state of Georgia alone it is estimated that there are 45,000 teenage alcoholics and approximately the same number of young problem drinkers (Kalber, 1981).

AREAS OF RESEARCH

There are basically five areas of research that explore variables influencing adolescent drinking: (1) parental influence, (2) peer influence, (3) environmental influence, (4) psychological variables, and (5) adolescents' attitudes toward alcohol. It is recognized that the prevalence of alcohol consumption among high school students is the result of development through predictable channels of imitation, identification, and role modeling of significant others in the person's environment (U.S. Department of Health and Human Services, 1981; U.S. Department of Health, Education and Welfare, 1971, 1974). This manuscript reviews these areas and subsequently elaborates the rationale for the intervention model chosen. It concludes with a discussion of the evaluation of the model.

Effective, comprehensive methods of teaching pupils about alcohol must be found if the youths are to make well-informed decisions about drinking. To have a full impact on youths, such education should be presented in the early adolescent years, following the influence of the parental/home setting and coinciding with the influx of the peer influence. This stage usually begins at ages 12 or 13, most often in the seventh and eighth grades. By age 15, many adolescents are drinking heavily (U.S. Department of Health and Human Services, 1981). If a program influences peer norms with a sociocultural approach, individuals can make knowledgeable, unpressured, personal decisions regarding the use of alcohol. This is crucial for this age group. Following the establishment of peer pressure to begin drinking, there is little chance of reconstituting the peer norms.

Adolescents spend approximately 50% of their waking hours in the school. School composes the society of youth—a society in which parents are excluded, the rulers are peers, and teachers at best play the role of consultants. It stands to reason therefore that the school might provide a viable conduit for relaying information about alcohol to adolescents. It is critical, however, that young adolescents are presented with alcohol education that is exciting, motivating, personalized, and nonjudgmental.

Unfortunately, the traditional classroom method using individual tasks and having students work alone toward a goal with few participatory, active learning experiences leads to competition for grades (Wodarski, 1981; Wodarski, Adelson, Tidball & Wodarski, 1980). At best, using this method with alcohol education could lead to little more than a push for a good grade. At worst, there could be classroom bravado leading toward reinforcement of tendencies *not* to learn about alcohol. Perhaps most unfortunate of all is the possibility of the class being split into the categories of high-performing students (by either teacher or student standards) and low-performing students who are often scorned.

An alternative to the traditional approach is one based on a behavioral group work perspective and encompassing peer support and group reward structures. Teams-Games-Tournaments (TGT) is an example of such an approach. TGT was developed through extensive research on games as teaching devices, using small groups as classroom work units, and emphasizing the task-and-reward structures used in the traditional classroom. The TGT technique is an alternative teaching approach that fully utilizes structure emphasizing group, rather than individual, achievement (Feldman & Wodarski, 1975; Wodarski, 1981; Wodarski et al., 1980).

There was evidence in field studies comparing TGT with traditional approaches to teaching in the third through the twelfth grades that students participating in TGT demonstrated higher academic achievement than did those in traditional settings. Moreover, TGT in many instances resulted in improved attitudes toward school, more peer tutoring, increased perceived probability of success, more social attachment to school and peers, and greater value attached by students to success in the classroom (DeVries & Slavin, 1978; Wodarski, 1981). On the basis of these positive results using TGT, it was posited that this technique would be successful in teaching youths about alcohol. The special timeliness of TGT in teaching adolescents about alcohol and how to make better decisions regarding its use is that TGT gives all students an equal opportunity to succeed. The students compete against teams whose members are at similar achievement levels. Points earned by low achievers are just as valuable to the overall team score as points earned by high achievers. This is in contrast to the typical instructional method that centers on individual assessment compared to the total class. Means of teaching low achievers are crucial, as low achievers are at greater risk than high achievers in regard to alcohol abuse (Wodarski & Lenhart, 1984). Thus, TGT's unique characteristic of motivating low achieving students increases the probability that students at high risk for alcohol abuse will receive the knowledge and be involved in a group process which reduces this risk.

METHOD

The following section provides a brief overview of an alcohol education program that is now being tested throughout the State of Georgia. The overview is followed by a more detailed outline of key facets of the program, including specific components, the dependent variables, and the evaluation procedures.

Prior to the implementation of the educational program, students complete the assessment instruments that compose the baseline data. These instruments are divided into three categories: (1) assessment of the student's knowledge of alcohol; (2) inventories designed to measure the student's attitudes about alcohol use, motivation and peer influence to drink, attitudes toward external control of alcohol consumption (such as legal or parental controls), knowledge of consequences of abuse, and discord in family relations; (3) self-inventories designed to measure current alcohol use and any current problem drinking behavior by students.

Five school systems are participating in the research. These school systems are located in metropolitan (1), semi-metropolitan (2), and rural (2) areas. Superintendents granted administrative approval for participation in the research and consent forms were obtained from all students. The participants underwent a four-week educational program that focused on alcohol information and the application of concepts to their own lives. The program emphasizes behavioral objectives through self-management skills that lead to responsible drinking practices.

TGT procedure. A 200-item pool of test items was developed according to the content contained within the curriculum. From this pool, 50 questions were randomly selected for both the pretest and posttest. The completion of the pretest of alcohol knowledge provided the basis for division of students into eight-member teams within each experimental classroom. The teams are organized into high achievers (those with a high level of knowledge concerning alcohol), middle achievers (those with moderate levels of knowledge), and low achievers (those most lacking in knowledge). Achievement scores for other areas of education are not used in compiling the team groups. The teams are heterogeneous, including two high achievers, four middle achievers, and two low achievers. Thus, the average achievement level is approximately equal across teams. The achievement levels of individual students are not revealed.

The alcohol education units are presented for fifty minutes each day for four weeks. The first three days of each week are devoted to learning alcohol concepts through discussions and various participatory activities. The fourth day focuses on working in the TGT teams on worksheets in preparation for the tournament, which is held on the fifth day of each week.

The tournament games consist of short-answer questions designed to assess and reinforce the knowledge gained in class. These are played by team members individually competing against other team members of comparable achievement levels. The team members are assigned to a tournament table where they compete against three students of comparable achievement levels from other teams. Scores are kept for each individual during the tournament games. At the end of the tournament, the top, middle, and low scorers at each table are awarded a fixed number of points for their teams.

The points earned by a student determine whether he or she will stay at the same tournament table or be moved to a table with higher- or lower-performing students for the next tournament. In this way, competitors change regularly, and the competition is not skewed in favor of any group of achievers. The points earned by an individual are added to those earned by other team members to compose a total team score. Teachers tabulate individual and team scores at the end of each tournament, and scores are posted the next school day.

The program of comprehensive alcohol education is comprised of the following:[1] *Alcohol Education*. The educational unit is in two parts. The first covers the biological, psychological, and sociocultural determinants of alcoholism. It is crucial that in learning about alcohol participants become informed of the multiple factors that have been shown to contribute to irresponsible use of alcohol and to alcoholism. This serves to assist them in making realistic judgments about their own present or possible future alcohol use and to inform them of the progression from responsible consumption, to problem usage, to alcoholism. This aspect of the program serves not as a scare tactic but is a research-based approach to what is currently known about the determinants of alcoholism.

The second and larger educational component consists of basic knowledge about alcohol consumption and usage. Students learn the gamut of topics related to the use of alcohol, including how much alcohol a body can absorb in a given length of time, when an intoxicated person is in an emergency situation and how to deal with such an occurrence, the physiological attributes of alcohol, the amount of alcohol in a variety of alcoholic beverages, and how to assess a drinking problem. Specific curriculum topics included are (1) Alcohol and Our Society, (2) What is Alcohol, (3) Short Term Effects of Alcohol: Intoxication and Hangover, (4) Values Clarification and Drinking, (5) Common Motivations for Drinking and Driving Behavior, (6) Drinking and Effects on Driving, (7) Alternatives to Drinking and Drinking-Driving in our Society, (8) Long Term Effects of Alcohol, and (9) Recognizing and Treating Drinking Problems.

Both divisions of the alcohol educational unit are taught via group discussions, participatory activities, and the TGT tournaments. All activities emphasize the use of peer support to enhance learning and the acceptance of responsible attitudes toward drinking.

Self-management. From the perspective of the self-management of one's lifestyle, students are taught basic principles of social learning theory related to alcohol consumption. Emphasis is placed on the theory that all drinking patterns — whether intelligent, abusive, or alcoholic — are learned. An individual with a drinking problem can learn to drink differently, and the drinker who currently has no problem can control circumstances so that his or her drinking will remain within acceptable bounds (Williams & Long, 1979).

Social learning theorists emphasize that the abuse of alcohol is learned from the consequences that follow drinking. These most often include (1) stress reduction, (2) removal from an unpleasant situation, and (3) an excuse for otherwise unacceptable behavior. There are many other potential reinforcers for alcohol abuse: peer pressure to drink and subsequent reinforcement by significant peers, having fun equated with how much one drinks, and the need to escape from thought of academic failure (Ali-brandi, 1978).

A fundamental theme is that students can change or determine behavior by altering the environment, be it internal or external. The two major categories of environmental events that must be understood and manipulated to produce the desired outcome are: events that precede and set the stage for particular behavior, and events that follow the behavior and make them more or less likely to occur (Williams & Long, 1979). Thus, one learning experience is to help students identify environmental events controlling behavior and then alter the ones necessary to produce the desired behavior. Examples of external environmental stimuli that cue drinking behavior are parties or peer statements. Examples of internal environmental events are emotional upset and loneliness. Students are instructed in how to remove or reduce stress-producing cues from the environment and how to engage in rewarding activities other than the consumption of alcohol.

A necessary aspect of self-management is learning to be assertive with others. Recent research has shown that young adult problem drinkers often feel dissatisfaction with their interpersonal relationships with others and perceive themselves as lacking in social skills.

The students learn how to cope with the task of interacting with others in a meaningful and satisfying way. Facets of the program developed by Lange and Jakubowski (1976) are used, including conversational skills training, use of appropriate nonverbal communication, and development of assertive behavior in learning to decrease stress produced by inadequately met social needs. Specific elements emphasized are: (1) how to introduce oneself, (2) how to initiate and continue conversations, (3) how to give and receive compliments, (4) how to enhance appearance, (5) how to make and refuse requests, (6) how to express feelings spontaneously, (7) how to use appropriate nonverbal behavior in enhancing sociability with others, (8) how to reward oneself for not drinking, and (9) how to have a helpful discussion with a significant other who has a drinking problem.

Role-play simulation exercises are used to help students practice refusing alcohol in a socially acceptable manner within normal peer contexts. This aspect of the program is modeled after the work of Foy and his associates (1976). General procedures are referred to as drink refusal training. The basic aim is to help students develop more effective ways of dealing with social pressures to consume alcohol. Specific situations are practiced in which individuals apply pressure to persuade others to consume excessive amounts of alcohol. Students practice reactions to statements such as "One drink won't hurt you," "What kind of friend are you?" or "Just have a little one, I'll make sure you won't have any more." Appropriate reactions are taught such as to (1) look directly at the pusher when responding, (2) speak in a firm, strong tone with appropriate facial expressions and body language, (3) offer an alternative suggestion such as "I don't care for a beer but I'd love a soft drink," (4) request that the pushers refrain from continued persuasion, or (5) change the subject. These areas of self-management skills are taught through group discussion and participatory activities and, when appropriate, are incorporated into the TGT tournaments.

Adolescents also may need training in terms of coping with daily academic and social problems. In such cases they are taught a problem-solving approach based on the work of D'Zurilla and Goldfried (1971), Goldfried and Goldfried (1975), Sarason and Sarason (1981), and Spivack and Shure (1974). The general components of these programs emphasize: (1) how to generate information; (2) how to generate possible solutions; (3) how to evaluate possible courses of action; (4) how to choose and implement strategies; and (5) verification of the outcomes of selected courses of action. Problem-solving strategies include: (1) explanation of how certain consequences and stimuli can control problem-solving behavior; (2) isolation and definition of the behaviors to be changed; (3) use of stimulus control techniques to influence rates of problem-solving behavior; and (4) use of appropriate consequences to either increase or decrease a behavior.

Instructor training. The sessions are led by the regular classroom teacher. The teachers are trained to talk comfortably with students about this sensitive issue, to be supportive of the group process, to have a sound knowledge base in social learning principles so as to help identify and analyze behavior, and to have complete and thorough knowledge of the TGT technique. Initially, teachers receive pertinent reading materials on the TGT technique, alcohol and alcohol abuse, and behavioral and self-management techniques. They are then trained by the researchers in the use of the curriculum and behavioral techniques. After the initial 4-hour training workshop the author was available to the teachers as a consultant. Periodic videotaping of the instructors leading a class was used to assure the proper level of competence in the implementation of the program.

Outcome Measures. The following scales and inventories were administered to all participants to provide baseline data on dependent variables. Subsequent measures of the phenomena will be obtained at posttesting and follow-up.

1. Knowledge of alcohol. This scale is based on information and myths about alcohol from Engs's (1977) scale. It also provided a portion of the material used to make up the TGT tournament quizzes.
2. Stumphauzer's (1980) "Behavioral Analysis Questionnaire for Adolescent Drinkers" is used for self-reports of drinking behavior. This scale is a twenty-item questionnaire that has been used to study the social learning variables in adolescents' alcohol use.
3. "The Adolescent Alcohol Questionnaire" by Glikson and associates (1980) is used to measure attitudes, motivation, and behavior associated with adolescents' alcohol use and abuse.
4. The "Index of Self-Esteem" and the "Generalized Contentment Scale" are used to provide information on students' psychosocial characteristics that could influence the tendency to drink (Hudson, 1982; Hudson & Proctor, 1977). Self-concepts and general satisfaction with life are assessed, which could be useful in future program planning.
5. The "Index of Family Relations" is used to measure the magnitude of problems that are found in family members' relationships (Hudson, Acklin & Bartosh, 1980).
6. The "Survey of Behavior" is used to measure a child's self-reports on level of impulsivity (Hollender, 1974).

Through these self-inventories and assessment tools, it is determined if students lack an awareness of alcohol issues. More importantly, those with a serious drinking problem are identified. When this occurs, the student is referred to the appropriate professional service outside the auspices of this program.

Follow-up. Follow-up of the program participants will be conducted for two years after completion of the educational program. The assessment scales used at pre- and posttest will be used at each follow-up interval to provide comparative data. In this way, maintenance of knowledge and behavior may be determined.

RESULTS

In all participating schools, students received either instruction according to the experimental TGT method, traditional instruction, or no instruction. In total, 570 participated in the experimental TGT procedure, 384 in traditional instruction, and 411 in a control or no-treatment condition. Four percent were seniors, 21% were juniors, 49% sophomores, and 27% freshmen.

Description of Drinking Behaviors

In our sample, 60% of the students indicated that they started to drink because they liked the taste; 18.2% said they wanted to be like their friends, and 13.6% said that it helped them to feel less nervous and tense. They drink a variety of intoxicants— 43.8% drink beer, 29.7% drink wine, 23.4% drink hard liquor, and 3.1% drink substitutes for alcohol such as cough medicine, mouth wash, and hair tonic. Of our student population, 21% received their drinks from parents or relatives, 54.5% from friends, 12.2% from their home without their parents' knowledge, and 9.8% from brothers or sisters. Only 2.4% buy liquor with a false identification.

Of our sample, 10.9% had their first drink before the age of 10, 21.9% had the first drink between the ages of 10 and 13, and 19.7% between the ages of 14 and 15. Thus, by the age of 15, 51.5% of our sample had already taken its first drink. Almost half (49.3%) of our students indicated that the reason they had their first drink was curiosity, 23.1% because parents or relatives offered it, and 10.4% to get drunk or high. Fifty-two percent drink with their friends their own age, while 13.8% drink with older friends. Thus peers are involved in drinking behaviors in about 66% of the situations, while only 21.5% drink with their parents.

The greatest effect from alcohol, it appears, is its ability to make the teenager feel loose and easy (52.2% response). In terms of ultimate effect, 16.8% get moderately high, 10.6% became drunk, 9.7% drink so heavily that they do not remember what happened the next day, 5.3% become ill, and the same percentage pass out. When asked, "What is the greatest effect that drinking has had on your life," 79.5% indicated no effect, 7.9% indicated that it has gotten them into trouble, 6.6% reported that it has interfered with having a good time and with school work, and 2.6% stated that it interfered with their relating with someone.

When asked how do others see them, most teenagers (84.9%) relate that others do not think that they have a problem, while 6.7% indicate that family or friends have advised them to control or to cut down on their drinking.

Out of a possible 19 reasons they could choose as reasons they drink they ranked the following highest:

    — to celebrate
    — I like the taste
    — it makes me feel good
    — it helps me relax
    — to liven up things when they are dull
    — to see how it will affect me

Alcohol Knowledge

Data in Figure 1 compare the amount of learning according to each group. The experimental classes had significant increases in knowledge about alcohol as compared to traditional and no instruction control groups ($F = 7.21$; $df = 2, 1347$; $p < .05$). School effects were not significant ($F = .59$; $df = 4, 1347$; $p > .05$). Thus the data are not confounded by particular characteris-

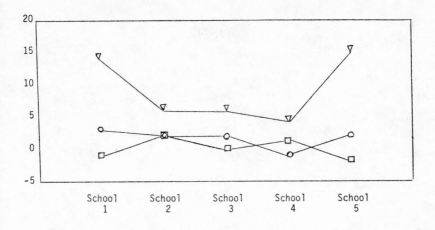

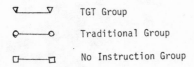

TGT Group

Traditional Group

No Instruction Group

Figure 1. Amount of learning according to social learning, traditional and no instruction groups and school.

tics of a school system. The increases between pre and posttest were as follows for the experimental groups: School 1, +14; School 2, +6; School 3, +6; School 4, +4; School 5, +15; with the average nonweighted mean being 9. This can be compared with the changes in the traditional instructional groups: School 1, +3; School 2, +2; School 3, +2; School 4, -1; School 5, +2; with the average nonweighted mean being 2.2. The changes in the no instructional groups were as follows: School 1, -1; School 2, +2; School 3, 0; School 4, +1; School 5, -2; with the average nonweighted mean being 0. The data suggest that the TGT procedure helps students gain knowledge about alcohol and effects on driving behaviors.

Data from the Engs Alcohol Knowledge Test which contains 36 true-false items, confirm our own measures of alcohol knowledge acquisition. Data in Table 1 show that our experimental

Table 1

Amount of Learning by School According to Social Learning, Traditional, and No Instruction Groups According to the Engs Alcohol Knowledge Inventory

	Type of Group					
	Social Learning		Traditional		No Instruction	
School	Pretest	Posttest	Pretest	Posttest	Pretest	Posttest
1	18	25	19	21	17	17
2	16	22	16	15	15	16
3	19	26	15	17	20	21
4	17	23	17	18	18	17
5	18	27	17	20	17	10
	88	123	84	91	87	90
	17.6	24.6 + 7*	16.8	18.2 + 1.4	17.4	18 + .6

* p < .05

groups increased 7 points, from a pretest average of 17.6 to 24.6. Our regular instructional groups increased from 16.8 to 18.2, an increase of 1.4. Our control groups that received no instruction increased from 17.4 to 18.0, an increase of .6. The differences between the experimental and both control groups are significantly different (F = 10.91; df 2, 1347; p < .05). Thus two different measures confirm the ability of the teams, games, and tournaments procedure to help students acquire knowledge about alcohol.

Drinking Behavior

As indicated in Table 2, students showed a substantial decrease in drinking behavior for the experimental procedure. Of the 6 items measured on a five-graded scale of the Engs inventory which assesses consumption, the experimental groups showed a 6.64 point change as compared to the .57 change in traditional instruction groups and a .49 change in the control groups. Higher scores indicate a decrease in the consumption of alcohol. The results between the experimental and the two other groups are significantly different (F = 8.89, df 2, 1347; p < .05).

The amount of alcohol consumed also favored the experimental groups as compared to the traditional and no instructional groups. Change from pre- to posttest on the amount of drinking by students revealed that the experimental group decreased 12.7% while the traditional instructional group and the control groups showed no reduction at all. The experimental group also had a significant reduction in the amount of alcohol consumed at any one session. The experimental group reduced the amount consumed at any one session by about 40%, compared to almost no reduction for the traditional instructional group or the control procedure. The experimental group increased almost 15 percentage points in regard to time elapsed from their last drink. Relatively no change occurred in the traditional and control groups. Students in the TGT group also showed changes in the time of day when they were drinking as compared to the traditional instructional group and the no instructional group. The most significant decrease for the TGT students occurred at night where they

Table 2

Amount of Change in Drinking Patterns as Assessed by the Engs Questionnaire (Items 1-6) According to the

Social Learning, Traditional, and No Instruction Groups

	Type of Group								
	Social Learning			Traditional			No Instruction		
Item	Pretest	Posttest	Change	Pretest	Posttest	Change	Pretest	Posttest	Change
1	1.48	2.58	+1.1	1.56	1.69	+.13	1.48	1.52	+.04
2	1.87	2.91	+1.04	1.77	1.89	+.12	1.57	1.59	+.02
3	1.63	2.73	+1.0	1.90	2.00	+.10	1.78	1.89	+.11
4	1.88	2.77	+.89	1.72	1.89	+.17	1.67	1.72	+.05
5	1.55	2.97	+1.42	1.63	1.78	+.15	1.55	1.72	+.17
6	1.87	2.96	+1.09	1.92	1.82	-.10	1.81	1.91	+.10
	10.28	16.92	+6.64*	10.52	11.07	+.57	9.86	10.35	+.49

* $p < .05$

reduced their drinking by one-third. Our data also indicate that the TGT students increased in self-confidence about their drinking behavior as compared to our traditional instruction and control group. (See Table 3.)

In regard to the adverse consequences of drinking, the Engs inventory revealed a significantly increased score (from 32.14 to 50.93 for the TGT groups; F = 14.11; df 2, 1347; p< .05). The other two groups had relatively no change. The differences between TGT and the two groups are significant. This indicates that students not only reduce the amount of alcohol they consumed but the consequences they suffered were reduced also.

Attitude Changes Concerning Drinking and Driving

The Drinking and Driving Questionnaire assessed attitude changes regarding drinking and driving behavior (Vegega, 1983). Twenty-three (23) items contained on the questionnaire relate to the specific effects of drinking and driving. For the experimental group, a significant positive (16.48) attitude change occurred. For the traditional instruction group the change was 2.68, and for the control group the change was .94. The TGT group was significantly different from the others (F = 12.88; df 2, 1347; p < .05).

Table 3

Amount of Change in Adversive Consequences from Drinking Behavior as Assessed by the Engs Questionnaire According to the Social Learning, Traditional, and No Instruction Groups

	Group		
	Social Learning	Traditional	No Instruction
Pretest	32.14	31.38	32.43
Posttest	50.93	32.43	34.11
Change	+18.79*	+.89	+1.68

p < .05

Nine items centered on the perception of being caught driving while drinking. The students believed that they had a one-in-two chance of being caught after drinking too much, and they felt that this was not high enough to deter them. They indicated that if the changes were 3-out-of-4 of getting caught, it would deter and/or stop them. They indicated that even if the police stopped them, the perceived chances of a negative consequence occurring were low — 1 in 3. They believed that the probability of consequences would have to be at least 3 in 4 in order to deter them from drinking. Thus, it is evident that the students perceived that the probability of being stopped by the police is low, and even if they are stopped by the police, the probability of subsequent application of negative consequences is also low.

Thirteen items dealt with ways of modifying their behavior in dealing with being too intoxicated. On these items, 7 significant differences occurred for the experimental group as compared to the traditional and no instruction group. Thus, the data indicate that TGT did have an effect on students' cognitive acquisition of behavioral options. (See Table 4.)

Related Assessment Techniques

The "Survey of Behavior" inventory indicated that the experimental groups became less impulsive; the change was 10.64 as compared to the traditional groups which changed 1.33 and no instruction group with a 2.78 change (Hollender, 1974). (See Table 5.) The changes for the TGT groups as compared to traditional and no instruction groups are statistically significant ($F = 14.87$; df 2, 1347; $p < .05$). Additionally, the TGT students experienced statistically significant increases in their feelings of self-esteem as measured by the "Index of Self-Esteem," and their peer relations as measured by the "Index of Peer Relations," as compared to traditional and no instruction groups (Hudson, 1982). Since our program addressed these aspects, the changes were expected. The TGT groups related no better to their families than did the traditional and no instruction groups as measured by the "Index of Family Relations."

Table 4

Significant and Nonsignificant Differences Between Experimental and Traditional
and No Instruction Control Groups in Perceived Means of Avoiding Driving After
Drinking Too Much

Item

Significant	Nonsignificant

1. Limiting my alcohol level by scheduling my drinks (e.g., every other drink nonalcoholic, drink more slowly).

2. Limiting my alcohol level by stopping my drinking at a predetermined time.

3. After I stop drinking, I wait until my alcohol level is "safe" for driving.

4. Asking someone else for a ride home.

5. Having one person volunteer not to drink in order to drive others home.

6. Offering to drive friends/guests home.

7. Avoid Situations where I know I tend to drive after drinking.

8. Intervene to stop a person from driving after drinking too much.

1. Having hosts/hostesses watch and schedule the drinking of guests.

2. Testing myself for my alcohol level (e.g., using a breath device, doing dexterity test).

3. Do not drink alcoholic beverages when I have to drive.

4. Call a taxi so that a friend/ guest will not drive after drinking too much.

5. Plan to stay overnight somewhere.

Table 5

Amount of Self-Reported Change in Impulsive Behavior According to Social Learning, Traditional, and No Instruction Groups

	Group		
	Social Learning	Traditional	No Instruction
Pretest	58.21	59.11	56.17
Posttest	47.57	57.78	53.39
Change	+10.64*	+1.33	+2.78

*$p < .05$

Teacher Evaluations

Teachers basically like the total curriculum and plan to use it next year. Moreover, they have expressed interest in expanding the TGT method to other subjects, particularly drugs. The major factor contributing to success appeared to be the self-contained nature of the curriculum guide. After implementation of the 4-week program, teachers realized that far too little time had been devoted previously to the topic.

Student Evaluations

The students enjoyed the TGT procedure compared to the traditional instruction and no instruction control groups. In particular, they liked working together in groups, the worksheets, and the tournaments. The majority (56%) of students in the TGT groups believed that they learned a lot about alcohol, compared with 30% in the traditional group and 29% in the control groups. More important, 86% of the TGT students believed that what they learned would affect how they drink in the future, compared to 60% in the traditional instruction and 55% in the no instruction groups. Ninety-six percent (96%) of the TGT students felt they knew what responsible drinking is after the completion of the TGT method, compared to only 67% of those in the traditional method and 30% in the control condition.

Additionally, students in the experimental group underwent a significant attitude change toward providing more alcohol education in the schools. Ideas mentioned included that programs should provide methods to resist peer pressure and alternatives to drinking, that alcohol education should occur early in the school, that alcohol education will influence their drinking habits, that the police should enforce DUI laws, and that advertisers should not link sex with drinking.

Significance

The TGT program is conceptualized to be an effective, thorough, and easy-to-administer vehicle by which to educate youth about alcohol and its effects on driving behavior. Moreover, it is believed to contribute to the development of responsible attitudes toward the use of alcoholic beverages. There are substantial practical, educational and methodological gains from this study. The program's unique combination of the presentation of educational materials in a manner which encourages peer support, and using a group reward structure and participatory learning, provide for the development of a new concept in teaching adolescents about alcohol.

The TGT technique has been shown to be effective in educating adolescents in the areas of nutrition, math, social studies, English, and so forth, as well as in increasing the value attached by students to success in the classroom. Its use in the acquisition of knowledge about alcohol, however, had not heretofore been tested. These data suggest that the TGT technique is effective in teaching adolescents about alcohol, a subject which is espoused to be of great importance but struggled with in terms of its presentation. Moreover, self-reports of TGT groups showed a lowered consumption of alcohol, a change in attitudes toward drinking and driving, and the acquisition of alternative behaviors for avoiding driving after drinking too much.

Of the most outstanding gains from this project is the development of an alcohol education program, complete with curriculum and explanation of educational techniques, that may be given to teachers who in turn can incorporate the units in their teaching with minimal additional training. Thus, in addition to providing valuable and essential descriptive data about adolescents' use and views about alcohol, and data reflective of effective methods to teach youth about alcohol, the project provides a complete educational package for further use by teachers and/or other school professionals. This allows teachers without formal training to easily implement an alcohol education unit.

It is widely agreed among experts in the area of alcoholism that the use of alcohol by adolescents has reached proportions of alarming concern. Unless effective programs are developed and implemented to assist youth in acquiring knowledge about alcohol and consequences of usage, the number of problem drinkers will continue to rise. Students and teachers alike have expressed need and interest in receiving training and education in this area. Yet, despite the widespread concern over the physical, social, and emotional consequences of adolescent alcohol abuse, there have been very few scientifically supported alcohol education programs (Reed, 1981).

The continued development and implementation of the program described here will provide an educational tool for increasing the likelihood of responsible decisions about alcohol use, especially as it relates to driving behavior. This is accomplished through the use of peer support, group rewards, knowledge, and practice of requisite behaviors for reducing the consumption of alcohol. Follow-up studies currently in progress will assess the long-term effects of the program on student knowledge, consumption of alcohol and attitudes toward drinking and driving.

NOTES

1. For an elaboration of the curriculum see Wodarski, J. S. & Lenhart, S. D. (1982). *Alcohol education by the team-games-tournaments method*. 2nd ed.; Minneapolis, MN: Burgess Publishing Company. A copy of the TGT training manual can be obtained by contacting the author at the following address: Dr. John S. Wodarski, Director, University of Georgia, School of Social Work Research Center, Tucker Hall, Athens, Georgia 30602.

REFERENCES

Abelson, H. I. (1977). *A national survey on drug use*. Rockville, MD: National Institute on Drug Abuse.
Alibrandi, T. (1978). *Young alcoholics*. Minneapolis, MN: CompCare Publications.

DeVries, S. & Slavin, R. (1978). Teams-games-tournaments (TGT): Review of 100 classroom experiments. *Journal of Research and Development in Education, 12*, 28-38.

D'Zurilla, T. J. & Goldfried, M. R. (1971). Problem solving and behavior modification. *Journal of Abnormal Psychology, 78*, 107-126.

Engs, R. C. (1977). Drinking patterns and drinking problems of college students. *Journal of Studies on Alcohol, 38*, 2144-2156.

Feldman, R. A. & Wodarski, J. S. (1975). *Contemporary approach to group treatment*. San Francisco, CA: Jossey-Bass.

Foy, C. W., Miller, P. M., Eisler, R. M. & O'Toole, O. H. (1976). Social skills training to teach adolescents to refuse drinks effectively. *Journal of Studies on Alcohol, 37*(9), 1340-1345.

Glikson, L., Smythe, P. C., Gorman, J. & Rush, B. (1980). The adolescent alcohol questionnaire: Its development and psychometric evaluation. *Journal of Drug Education, 10*(3), 209-227.

Goldfried, M. & Goldfried, A. (1975). Cognitive change methods. In F. Kanfer & A. Goldstein (Eds.), *Helping people change*. New York: Pergamon Press.

Hollender, J. W. (1976). The development of questionnaire measures of impulsivity. Unpublished manuscript, Emory University, Atlanta, Georgia. Cited in Johnson (Ed.), *Tests & measurements in child development: Handbook II*. San Francisco, CA: Jossey-Bass, p. 1168.

Hudson, W. W. (1982). *The clinical measurement package*. Homewood, IL: Dorsey Press.

Hudson, W. W., Acklin, J. D. & Bartosh, J. C. (1980). Assessing discord in family relationships. *Social Work Research & Abstracts, 16*, 21-29.

Hudson, W. W. & Proctor, E. K. (1977). Assessment of depressive affect in clinical practice. *Journal of Consulting and Clinical Psychology, 45*, 1206-1207.

Johnson, P. (1977). *U.S. adult drinking practices: Time trends, social correlates and sex roles* (draft report prepared for the National Institute on Alcohol Abuse and Alcoholism under contract no. ADM 281-76-0020). Santa Monica, CA: Rand Corp.

Kalber, E. (1981). Treatment of youth users criticized. *Athens, Georgia Banner Herald*, December 2, 1; 14.

Lange, A. J. & Jakubowski, P. (1976). *Responsible assertive behavior*. Champaign, IL: Research Press.

Rachal, J. V., Maisto, S. A., Guess, L. L. & Hubbard, R. L. (1982). *Alcohol use among adolescents* (Alcohol and Health Monograph 1, U.S. Department of Health and Human Services ADM 82-1190). Washington, DC: U.S. Government Printing Office.

Reed, D. S. (1981). Reducing the costs of drinking and driving. In M. Moore & D. Gerstein (Eds.), *Alcohol and public policy: Beyond the shadow of prohibition*. Washington, DC: National Academy Press.

Sarason, I. G. & Sarason, B. R. (1981). Teaching cognitive and social skills to high school students. *Journal of Consulting and Clinical Psychology, 49*(6), 908-919.

Spivack, G. & Shure, M. B. (1974). *Social adjustment of young children*. San Francisco, CA: Jossey-Bass.

Stumphauzer, J. S. (1980). Behavioral analysis questionnaire for adolescent drinkers. *Psychological Reports, 47*, 641-642.

U.S. Department of Health and Human Services (1981). *Fourth special report to the U.S. Congress on alcohol and health from the secretary of Health and Human Services* (DHHS Publication No. ADM 81-1080). Washington, DC: U.S. Government Printing Office.

U.S. Department of Health, Education and Welfare (1974). *Second special report to the U.S. Congress on alcohol and health from the secretary of HEW* (DHEW Publication No. HSM 72-9099). Washington, DC: U.S. Government Printing Office.

Vegega, M. E. (1983). *Reducing alcohol-impaired driving: Surveys for use in measuring program effectiveness*. Washington, DC: U.S. Department of Transportation, National Highway Traffic Safety Administration.

Williams, R. L. & Long, J. D. (1979). *Toward a self-managed lifestyle*. Boston, MA: Houghton Mifflin Co.

Wodarski, J. S. (1981). *The role of research in clinical practice*. Baltimore, MD: University Park Press.

Wodarski, J. S. & Lenhart, S. D. (1984). Alcohol education for adolescents. *Social Work Education, 6*(2), 69-92.

Wodarski, L. A., Adelson, C. L., Tidball, M. T. & Wodarski, J. S. (1980). Teaching nutrition by teams-games-tournaments. *Journal of Nutrition Education, 12*(2), 61-65.

Unilateral Family Therapy with the Spouses of Alcoholics

Edwin J. Thomas
Cathleen Santa
Denise Bronson
Daphna Oyserman

SUMMARY. The design and development of a unilateral family therapy for alcohol abuse is reported from a study of 25 spouses. Subjects were recruited from newspaper advertisements in which spouses of partners who had a drinking problem and refused to enter treatment were solicited to receive free professional assistance. Treatment embraced treatment orientation, clinical assessment, spouse role induction, abuser-directed interventions, spouse-directed interventions, and maintenance. Results indicated that the unilateral treatment program can be implemented, the spouses of uncooperative alcohol abusers can be assisted to function as a positive rehabilitative influence with their alcoholic mates, and that important positive gains for the abusers and spouses can be achieved. It is concluded that the unilateral approach should be experimentally evaluated and, if results are favorable, applied with other populations.

The consequences of excessive drinking are well known and have been amply documented. By consuming alcohol in excess, the alcohol abuser harms his or her health, incurs large costs for society through loss of work, loss of efficiency, and greater likelihood of being in traffic accidents. In addition, the alcohol

---

The research reported in this paper was supported in part by Grant 1 RO1 AA04163-03 of the National Institute on Alcohol Abuse and Alcoholism, Edwin J. Thomas, Principal Investigator.

Requests for reprints should be sent to Edwin J. Thomas, School of Social Work, the University of Michigan, Ann Arbor, Michigan 48109.

abuser increases the likelihood of distressed family relationships, violence in the family, reduced family stability, and marital dissolution. Alcohol abuse is clearly a difficult problem, but refusal of the abuser to enter treatment makes an already difficult problem worse. The alcohol abuser who refuses treatment poses troublesome and as yet unsolved problems concerning what the appropriate mode of treatment should be considering the needs of everyone involved.

There is an enormous population of individuals and families that potentially could benefit from intervention to reach the abuser. Writers have estimated that the combined remedial approaches to the alcohol problem reach no more than fifteen percent of the alcoholic population (Krimmel, 1971; Luks, 1983). This leaves an estimated 85 percent who are "hidden" and untreated excessive drinkers. If there are some ten million alcohol abusers (e.g., see Keller & Gurioli, 1976, and Steinglass 1976, for related estimates), there would be some 8.5 million who are thus "hidden." If one assumes further, as do Paolino and McCrady (1977), that for every alcohol abuser there are five other persons who suffer directly, this yields some 42.5 million individuals in the United States who could potentially benefit from improved or new methods of assistance that could reach them.

There is increasing evidence that the spouse, as a critical and sometimes sole point of leverage, may be used productively in rehabilitative efforts with alcohol-abusing partners. For example, the involvement of nonalcoholic wives in the treatment of their alcoholic husbands appears in some studies to be associated with relevant positive outcomes (e.g., Cadogan, 1973; Corder, Corder & Laidlaw, 1972; Ewing, Long & Wenzel, 1961; Gliedman, 1957; Hedberg & Campbell, 1974; McCrady, Paolino, Longabaugh & Rossi, 1979). Reports of efforts to work alone with the spouses of alcoholics indicate some benefits for the spouses (e.g., Cheek, Franks, Laucius & Burtle, 1971; Estes, 1977; Igersheimer, 1959). Some studies using selected confrontive tactics have described gains for the alcohol-abusing spouses as well (e.g., Hall, 1984; Howard & Howard, 1978; Johnson, 1973; Maxwell, 1976; Thorne, 1983; Zimberg, 1982). However, to our knowledge, there has been no systematic evaluation of the effectiveness of these interventions. Particularly suggestive are analogous attempts to program wives to bring about changes for their spouses (e.g., Goldstein, 1971, as reported in Jacobson & Martin, 1976; Scheiderer & Bernstein, 1976; Szapocznik, Franks, Kurtines, Foote & Perez-Vidal, 1983), although the helping methodology in these efforts is not well developed for working with spouses in general nor was it used with spouses of alcohol abusers.

Up to this point, there has been no systematically developed and tested intervention methodology applicable to reaching cooperative spouses of uncooperative alcohol abusers. Al-Anon is a valuable alternative resource. However, by virtue of its lay and inspirational character and its requirement of anonymity, this self-help methodology cannot be adopted directly by alcohol counselors and other helping persons. Nor in the area of marital and family therapy is there a recognized unilateral approach to reach uncooperative members. The main emphasis in most family therapies is on the family as a system, in which treatment is best carried out with all or most family members. Treatment of the individual for marital and family distress is generally at best a minor variant, acknowledged by some writers as a particular format for marital and family therapy (e.g., Bennun, 1984; Carter & Orfanidis, 1976; Cookerly, 1976; Meeks & Kelly, 1970; Olson, 1975; Prochaska & Prochaska, 1978; Stahmann, 1977; Steinglass, 1978). There has been increasing emphasis upon family treatment approaches in the alcoholic marriage (e.g., Berenson, 1976; Bowen, 1974; Dulfano, 1978; Finlay, 1974; Jansen, 1977; Meeks & Kelly, 1970; Steinglass, 1976, 1978; Ward & Faillace, 1970), but there is no recognized unilateral family approach in the area of alcohol abuse. The use of family members in the alcohol area to confront the abuser to induce him to enter treatment is illustrated by the confrontive "intervention" of the Johnson approach (1973). It is valuable, but it represents only one of many alternatives that may be employed in a unilateral treatment with cooperative family members. Clearly, present intervention methods of alcohol counselors need to be augmented to reach and assist the uncooperative abuser and his or her spouse.

The purpose of this paper is to present an overview of a three-year pilot project to develop a unilateral family therapy for alcohol abuse. The main emphasis in this report is upon the treatment program that was developed.

THE CONCEPTION OF UNILATERAL FAMILY THERAPY

The design and development of the treatment program to reach the uncooperative alcohol abuser was guided by a working conception of unilateral family therapy (Thomas & Santa, 1982).

As a mode of family therapy, unilateral family therapy is intervention directed toward changing the behavior of an uncooperative family member through working with a cooperative member as mediator. As in family therapy in general, the unilateral approach also has the goals of altering individual difficulties that arise from family dynamics, improving interpersonal relationships in the family, and, in general, of enhancing family functioning. However, in the unilateral mode it is not possible to work with all or most members of the family as is usually the case in family therapy. Unilateral treatment is carried out with one or more cooperative family members without the direct involvement of one or more others who refuse to participate. This refusal to participate in treatment may be due to the family member's failure to recognize that a problem exists, lack of motivation to change, or both. Those family members who do participate may be clients in therapy as well as the mediators of change for the nonparticipating parties.

A major feature of the unilateral approach is a conception of the role of cooperative family member as client as well as mediator of change for the uncooperative family member. This emphasis does not assume that the cooperative member is to blame for the difficulties but rather that this person is a potentially crucial point of leverage whose strengths and influence may be productively employed in treatment to achieve change when other avenues of influence are limited or foreclosed. Thus, the spouse is viewed in the unilateral approach as a vital and potentially active agent of positive change who may be the main or only rehabilitative influence accessible to the practitioner.

There are three main foci of intervention in the unilateral approach. The first is the *individual focus* with emphasis on coping for the cooperative family member. When working with the spouse, such individual difficulties as stress, anxiety, lack of assertiveness, depression, anger, emotional overinvolvement, and failure to realize personal or career objectives could be the focus of intervention. The second is the *interactional focus* with emphasis predominantly upon family functioning. Among the areas of intervention for this focus are marital and family communication, decision making and conflict resolution, parent-child relationships, and sexual and affectional enhancement for the marital partners. The last is the *third party focus* which involves work with the spouse or other family member to bring about change for the uncooperative family member. Among the methods here are (a) inducing the uncooperative member to seek treatment or other assistance, (b) removing spouse, family or environmental conditions which serve to promote the problem behavior, and (c) providing support for non-problem behavior of the uncooperative member.

It is this combination of interventional foci along with working only with one or a few cooperative family members in a rehabilitative capacity that makes the unilateral approach a distinctive mode of therapy. Although considered here in terms of alcohol abuse, the unilateral approach has potential applicability to many other types of clientele not now accessible. Further details concerning the unilateral approach are to be found in Thomas and Santa (1982).

THE PROJECT

Overview

In keeping with the developmental objectives of the research, this pilot research placed primary emphasis on the design and development of a unilateral family therapy for alcohol abuse. Potential subjects were recruited from newspaper advertisements in which spouses of partners who had a drinking problem and refused to enter treatment were solicited to receive free professional assistance. Treatment was given by four clinician-researchers, consisting of the Project Director (E.J.T.), and three advanced doctoral students in the Doctoral Program in Social Work and Psychology who had MSW degrees and relevant clinical experience. Clinical and developmental effort for each case was carefully assessed, planned, supervised and monitored. Staff consultation was used for all major decisions.

The D&D Perspective

To meet objectives of design and development (D&D), cases were selected, as described below, to meet the criterion of developmental relevance; practice was conducted with D&D objectives as well as therapeutic aims; effort was evaluated at this early point in D&D largely in terms of the adequacy of the treatment methods being evolved; and the design for evaluation was selected to allow for D&D flexibility (for further details concerning developmental research and intervention design, see Thomas, 1984).

Eligibility Criteria

Cases were selected by criteria to assure their developmental relevance to the unilateral approach. Spouses making contact with the project were already solicited on the basis of their partner having a drinking problem and being unwilling to receive treatment for it. These were basic criteria for the abuser. Criteria for the spouse included recognition that the partner had a drinking problem, willingness to receive help to try to moderate the partner's drinking, and absence of a drinking problem for that spouse. Additional criteria for both marital partners were that there was no domestic violence, no other drug abuse, no history of severe emotional disorder, no immediate plans for marital dissolution, and that the partners were not then receiving professional counseling. These criteria served to keep the domain of D&D feasible and manageable.

Human subjects criteria for the abuser were provision of the abuser's consent to allow the spouse to disclose information about the abuser and to allow the spouse to try to facilitate the abuser's sobriety. For the non-alcohol abusing spouse, consent was obtained for the spouse to participate as a client in unilateral family therapy and to provide assessment information. These criteria were required by federal regulations for research with human subjects.

Subject Characteristics

A total of 25 spouses participated to varying degrees as subjects. The mean age of the spouses was 43 years, with 85% of them having had at least some college education. All but one spouse were white and all but one were female. Spouses had been married to abusers 15 years, on the average, and this was the first marriage for the majority. The only noteworthy difference for abusers was that they tended to be somewhat more educated than their spouses. Most participants had children living at home, typically one to three offspring. The median household income was reported to be in the $25,000 to $29,000 bracket. Nineteen of the spouses and 21 of the alcohol abusing partners were employed at the time of the initial assessment.

Available evidence from subjects who participated in assessment shows that the abusers indeed had a drinking problem. For example, in completing a spouse version of the Michigan Alcohol Screening Test to measure drinking behavior of the abuser, spouses produced average scores of 23 for the abuser. Spouses also reported that abusers consumed an average of 81.1 ounces per week of alcohol equivalent to 86 proof, and that all abusers were problem drinkers. Spouses and abusers participating in assessment reported that the abusers had been drinking at their present level for a mean of about eight years. Thirteen abusers participated in assessment and they had a mean MAST score of 18.1, considerably higher than the cut-off score of 5 which indicates there is an alcohol problem (Selzer, 1971).

Research Design

In keeping with the developmental objectives, a research design was adopted that allowed for clinical and developmental flexibility while also providing a basis for evaluation. The basic unit in the design was each pair of spouses who entered the project. One spouse in each successive pair was assigned at random to receive unilateral family therapy for six months, and the other spouse was assigned to a condition of delayed treatment. When therapy was terminated for the original unilateral therapy spouse, treatment was given to the delayed treatment spouse. D&D was conducted with four series, each having a relatively small number of spouses (Series I had 10 subjects and treatment lasted 6 months, Series II and III, both very brief special purpose series, had a total of 5 subjects, and Series IV had 10 subjects in which treatment lasted 4 months). A battery of some 20 assessment instruments was administered before and after treatment and at 6- and 12-month follow-ups. These included instruments to measure spouse coping (e.g., Life Distress Scale), family functioning (e.g., the Dyadic Adjustment Scale), and abuser drinking behavior (e.g., The Quantity-Frequency Schedule). Clinical assessment and monitoring were also carried out throughout treatment.

RESULTS

Given the D&D objectives of the research, the treatment program that evolved is necessarily a principal product. The results relating to the evaluation of outcomes were relevant but were secondary at this stage of development. Accordingly, an overview of the treatment program is presented below along with a summary of some of the quantitative outcomes relating to effectiveness.

The Treatment Program

Intervention in the unilateral mode, as described earlier, entails one or more of three possible foci. As applied to alcohol abuse, the individual focus involves the coping behavior of the cooperative nonalcohol abusing spouse, the interactional focus entails the marital and family functioning of that spouse, and the third-party focus emphasizes the drinking behavior of the uncooperative alcohol abuser. In the treatment program that evolved, the third-party focus was paramount, and the primary goal was to have the uncooperative abuser enter treatment for the alcohol abuse, or reduce the drinking through abstinence or (this failing) controlled drinking. To accomplish these objectives, abuser-directed interventions were carried out by the spouse serving as mediator of change for the abuser. The individual and interactional foci involved largely working with the spouse as mediator, where treatment was first directed toward induction of the spouse into the role of a positive rehabilitative agent as preparation for undertaking abuser-directed interventions mediated by the spouse.

Treatment embraced the following six areas: treatment orientation, clinical assessment, spouse role induction, abuser-directed interventions, spouse-directed interventions, and maintenance. Each of these is summarized below.

Treatment Orientation

Because the treatment program was new and differed considerably from most others, the treatment orientation was directed toward informing the spouse as fully as possible concerning what was in store for him or her. The spouse was prepared by explaining a number of points, such as the following: (a) the three foci of intervention, i.e., spouse coping, family functioning and sobriety facilitation; (b) the rights of the spouse to receive treatment and likewise the right of the abuser to refuse treatment; (c) the importance of keeping in confidence the matters discussed in the treatment; (d) the relationship between drinking behavior and family dynamics, with emphasis on the role of family factors in drinking behavior, the assumption that the spouse was not to be blamed for the excessive drinking of a partner, and the potential of the spouse to become a positive rehabilitative influence with the alcohol abuser; (e) the treatment regimen, including an overview of the main phases and an explanation of the importance of maintaining spouse input and cooperation in gathering data and formulating the intervention plan, not carrying out premature or ad hoc change efforts with the abuser, intervening only as planned with the therapist at the agreed upon time, and following the agreed upon plan as stipulated; and (f) the assurance that although some of the treatment methods were new and experimental and further research was needed to validate the approach, results to date had indicated that the approach could be implemented successfully in the majority of cases.

Clinical Assessment

Following the orientation, clinical assessment was conducted to obtain data from the spouse in areas such as the following: (a) factors affecting applicability and appropriateness of the unilateral approach, (b) abuser drinking patterns and history, (c) willingness of the abuser to seek treatment, (d) the abuser's capability to stop or reduce drinking, (e) increasers and decreasers of the abuser's drinking, (f) alternatives to drinking for the abuser, (g) the abuser's propensity toward physical violence, (h) interventional possibilities with the abuser, (i) spouse mediator capabilities, (j) areas in which the spouse may exercise influence and control with the abuser, (k) spouse conceptions of alcohol and alcohol abuse rehabilitation, (l) patterns of spouse enabling of the abuser's drinking, (m) possibilities to enhance the marital relationship, and (n) the characteristic ways in which the spouse has endeavored to change the abuser as part of the "old influence system." The information was obtained through interviews with the spouse and, where appropriate, by obtaining spouse recording of events outside the interview. Data such as these were then used to prepare an intervention plan.

Spouse Role Induction

Spouses were typically not ready at the beginning of treatment to serve as mediators of change for the abuser and to assume a positive rehabilitative role. Before abuser-directed interventions could be introduced, it was necessary to help the spouse adopt a positive rehabilitative role. Induction to change the role of the spouse was carried out independently from, and in advance of, endeavoring directly to alter the drinking behavior of the abuser. There were four modules involved in the role induction, each of which is briefly described below. Intervention in each of these areas was given, as needed, on an individual basis and not necessarily in the order indicated.

1. *Alcohol Education.* To counter misconceptions and misinformation concerning alcohol and its effects, alcohol education was given as necessary in such areas as: the nature and promise of contemporary treatment for alcohol abuse; the

characteristic behavior of alcohol abusers; the effects of alcohol; the seriousness of alcohol abuse for health, work performance, and family and psychological functioning; and the role of learning and family factors in excessive drinking.

2. *Enhancement of the Marital Relationship*. Since discordant marital relationships may impede efforts of the spouse to serve as the mediator of change, relationship enhancement was introduced to reduce the discord and conflict, to facilitate more harmonious marital relationships, and to potentiate the ability of the spouse to influence the abuser. Relationship enhancement consisted of interventions directed toward having the spouse carry out behaviors when the abuser was sober that the abuser would find enjoyable and that the spouse was willing and able to carry out. The objective was to improve marital relationships above current levels, given the motivation and capability of the spouse at that time.

3. *Disenabling*. To counter the ways in which the spouse enabled the abuser's drinking, a tailor-made program to reduce the enabling was introduced, with emphasis placed on the major areas in which the spouse had been enabling the abuser's drinking.

4. *Neutralizing the Old Influence System*. To diminish dysfunctional aspects of the "old influence system," such as nagging, complaining, and threatening, focus in this module was placed on neutralizing the customary and generally ineffective ways in which the spouse had endeavored to control the drinking of the abuser.

Abuser-Directed Intervention

The purpose of abuser-directed interventions was to induce the abuser to enter treatment for his or her alcohol abuse or to reduce the drinking, or both. The reduced drinking would ideally take the form of abstinence, but, in some cases, moderated drinking short of abstinence was the best outcome that could be achieved on a temporary basis, with abstinence being the final goal. Two intervention methods particularly appropriate for getting the abuser to enter treatment are given below:

1. *Programmed Confrontation of the Abuser*. The aim of programmed confrontation was to confront the abuser so that
he or she would be induced to enter treatment for the alcohol abuse and/or to decrease or stop drinking. Programmed
confrontations entailed training the spouse to confront the
abuser firmly but compassionately in the presence of the
therapist concerning the particulars and adverse effects of
the abuser's drinking; to present the abuser with specific
directives to enter treatment and/or to decrease or stop
drinking; and to present the consequences that the spouse
planned to carry out if the abuser failed to take the specified
action. What distinguishes programmed confrontation from
most confrontive interventions, including the Johnson
(1973) approach, to which it bears some similarities, is that
programmed confrontation involves systematic assessment,
intervention planning, implementation, and follow-up. Programmed confrontation is a powerful induction that can be
very successful providing that it is used with great care and
when selected conditions are met. Among the important
preconditions for using this intervention are that other interventional alternatives are not feasible and that the spouse is
willing to follow through with a strong consequence if the
recommended action is not taken.

2. *Programmed Request*. The programmed request consisted
of a carefully timed, staged and delivered request to have
the abuser carry out a recommended action, usually to enter
treatment for excessive drinking. The programmed request
requires as much planning and rehearsal as programmed
confrontation and, when appropriate, can be strong enough
to accomplish its objective. Among the conditions that need
to be met to implement a programmed request are some
readiness on the part of the abuser to respond favorably to
the request and unwillingness of the spouse to carry out a
strong consequence if the abuser fails to comply with the
request.

Additional abuser-directed interventions are particularly
appropriate for endeavoring to achieve the goal of reduced

drinking, whether or not the interventions above are employed or the abuser enters treatment. In each of these interventions, as with those described above, the spouse served as a mediator to carry out the intervention with the abuser, doing so on the basis of a treatment plan found to be feasible and appropriate in work with the therapist. There were four such interventions as follows:

3. *Spouse-Mediated Sobriety Facilitation*, which consisted of spouse behaviors that served to strengthen nondrinking alternatives for the abuser and to weaken abuser inducements to drinking;

4. *Programmed Self-Control*, which was directed toward helping the abuser achieve self-control of his or her own drinking behavior through mediation of the spouse;

5. *Programmed Decision Making*, which was decision making, instigated by the therapist through the spouse, directed toward having the marital partners reach a mutually satisfactory decision regarding the reduction of the abuser's drinking or of the conditions relating to such drinking; and

6. *Programmed Contingency Contracting*, which consisted of contingency contracts established between the spouse and the abuser directed toward achieving moderated drinking and/or entry into treatment for alcohol abuse. Each of these four interventions, like the programmed confrontation and programmed request, has particular conditions that make them the appropriate course of treatment.

Spouse-Directed Interventions

Although the main efforts of the unilateral approach are directed toward inducing the spouse to assume a positive rehabilitative role and on instigating abuser-directed interventions as described above, there are conditions under which interventions are directed expressly toward the spouse. One of these conditions is when an abuser-directed intervention has been employed without success, and it is no longer appropriate to try to change the abuser's drinking through the spouse or to get the abuser into treatment. Rather, the primary objective at this point is to improve the well being of the spouse.

In such instances, treatment may be oriented toward *disengaging*, which is focused on increasing the spouse's independence from the abuser and reducing his or her emotional involvement in the abuser's drinking problem. In addition to being something of a last resort, disengaging may sometimes be appropriate to combine with abuser-directed interventions, whether the abuser has entered treatment or has made improvement in reducing the drinking.

In addition to disengaging, *other interventions* used to assist the spouse to cope more effectively included working with such emotional problems and reactions of the spouse as stress, anxiety, lack of assertiveness, depression, and anger. These are addressed when removal of such difficulties may facilitate the therapist's work toward helping the spouse to bring about positive changes in the abuser's drinking behavior and improve his or her personal functioning.

Maintenance

Two additional interventions served to foster maintenance and generalization of the positive changes achieved and to help prevent relapse into excessive drinking. The first was *spouse support* to enable the spouse to continue to engage in the new behaviors after she or he had completed treatment and to help prevent the spouse from returning to previously maladaptive ways of behaving that might lessen her or his satisfaction with the marriage or threaten the abuser's sobriety.

The second intervention, *spouse-mediated relapse prevention training*, included the following areas as applied to the abuser: (a) identification of high risk situations for drinking, (b) temptation resistance training, (c) acceleration of nondrinking behaviors, (d) handling of relapses, (e) education concerning the nature of relapses and how they may be prevented, and (f) restoration of balance in life style, (e.g., see Gordon & Marlatt, 1981; Marlatt, 1982).

Each of the interventions described above was applied on an individual basis after assessment had been completed and the intervention in question had been found to be appropriate and feasible. The duration of treatment was generally four to six months (depending upon the series the spouse was in), sometimes less if the treatment goals for the abuser had been achieved.

OUTCOME RESULTS

The effects of treatment were analyzed within the limitations of the number of subjects. There was a maximum of 25 spouses available for analysis, 15 of whom received treatment in either Series I or Series IV for a period of 4 to 6 months. Of these 15, 9 received immediate treatment and 6 received delayed treatment. Of the 10 subjects who were classified in the nontreatment category, 3 had no contact with the project for purposes of treatment, 2 had limited contact and an additional 5 (from Series II and III) also had limited contact. Although the number of subjects in the categories was too small for conducting systematic statistical analysis, selected comparisons were made between the immediate and delayed treatment subjects and between all those who received treatment and those who did not.

There was a 53% reduction in alcohol consumption from before to after treatment for the abusers of spouses who received treatment, with a slight increase for the abusers of spouses who did not receive treatment. In a related analysis, all 13 subjects who received immediate or delayed treatment, for whom the relevant data were available, were classified in terms of whether there was improvement; the criterion for improvement was set at a reduction in drinking of 53% or more or entry into treatment, or both. Eight or 61% of the 13 abusers of spouses who had received treatment improved, whereas none of the 6 abusers of spouses improved who did not receive treatment ($p = .02$ by Fisher's Exact Test).

Repeated measures analyses of variance were also conducted in which the effects of immediate treatment were contrasted with those of delayed treatment and the combined treatment subjects were contrasted with those for nontreatment. It was found that treatment was clearly associated with a reduction in drinking behavior and a diminution of general life distress. Some positive gains were also evident for affectional expression and sexual satisfaction for the marital partners. These areas of positive change tended to be those that were targeted in treatment, particularly the drinking behavior. There were no other positive changes for other areas, and there were no statistically significant negative changes for any of the variables analyzed. A detailed report of the quantitative results will be presented elsewhere.

CONCLUSION

Considered altogether, the results of the research indicate that the unilateral treatment program can be implemented, the spouses of uncooperative alcohol abusers can be assisted to function as a positive rehabilitative influence with their alcohol abusing mates, and that important positive gains for the abusers and spouses can be achieved. Positive changes were found in the analyses of outcomes in spite of the small number of subjects and the fact that the treatment program was in the process of development. These results confirm the promise of the unilateral approach and highlight the importance of conducting systematic experimental evaluation. If such inquiry yields additional favorable findings, the unilateral approach should be applied with other populations of alcohol abusers and other types of uncooperative and hard-to-reach family members.

REFERENCES

Bennun, I. (1984). Marital therapy with one spouse. In K. Hahlweg & N. S. Jacobson (Eds.), *Marital interaction: Analysis and modification*, pp. 356-374. New York: Guilford.

Berenson, D. (1976). A family approach to alcoholism. *Psychiatric Opinion, 13*, 33-38.

Bowen, M. (1974). Alcoholism as viewed through family systems theory and family psychotherapy. *Annals of the New York Academy of Science, 233*, 115-122.

Cadogan, D. A. (1973). Marital group therapy in the treatment of alcoholism. *Quarterly Journal of Studies in Alcohol, 34*, 1187-1194.

Carter, E. & Orfanidis, M. M. (1976). Family therapy with one person and the family therapists's own family. In P. J. Guerin (Ed.), *Family therapy: Theory and practice*. New York: Garner Press.

Check, F. E., Franks, C. M., Laucius, J. & Burtle, V. (1971). Behavior modification training for wives of alcoholics. *Quarterly Journal of Studies on Alcohol, 32*, 456-461.

Cookerly, J. R. (1975). Evaluating different approaches to marriage counseling. In D. H. L. Olson (Eds), *Treating relationships*. Lake Mills, IA: Graphic Publishing Co.

Corder, B. F., Corder, R. F. & Laidlaw, N. L. (1972). An intensive treatment program for alcoholics and their wives. *Quarterly Journal of Studies on Alcohol, 33*, 1144-1146.

Dulfano, C. (1978). Family therapy of alcoholism. In S. Zimberg, J. Wallace & S. B. Blume (Eds.), *Practical approaches to alcoholism psychotherapy*. New York: Plenum Press.

Estes, N. J. (1977). Counseling the wife of an alcoholic spouse. In N. J. Estes & M. E. Heinemann (Eds.), *Alcoholism: Development, consequences and interventions*. St. Louis: Mosby.

Ewing, J. A., Long, V. & Wenzel, G. G. (1961). Concurrent group psychiatric treatment of alcoholic patients and their wives. *International Journal of Group Psychotherapy, 11*, 329-338.

Finlay, D. G. (1974). Alcoholism: Illness or problem in interaction? *Social Work, 19*, 398-405.

Gliedman, L. H. (1957). Concurrent and combined group therapy of chronic alcoholics and their wives. *International Journal of Group Psychotherapy, 7*, 414-424.

Goldstein, M. K. (1971). Behavior rate change in marriages: Training wives to modify husbands' behavior. Doctoral Dissertation, Cornell University. *Dissertation Abstracts International, 23*, 548 (University Microfilms Number 71-17, 094).

Gordon, J. R. & Marlatt, G. A. (1981). Addictive behaviors. In J. R. Shelton & Rona L. Levy (Eds.), *Behavioral assignments and treatment compliance*. Champaign, IL: Research Press.

Hall, S. P. (1984). Training parents of adolescent drug and alcohol abusers as counselors. A symposium paper presented at the Association for Behavior Analysis Annual Meetings, Nashville, Tennessee.

Hedberg, A. G. & Campbell, L. (1974). A comparison of four behavioral treatments of alcoholism. *Journal of Behavior Therapy and Experimental Psychiatry, 5*, 251-257.

Howard, D. P. & Howard, N. T. (1978). Treatment of the significant other. In S. Zimberg, J. Wallace & S. B. Blume (Eds.), *Practical approaches to alcoholism psychotherapy*. New York: Plenum Press.

Igersheimer, W. W. (1959). Group psychotherapy for non-alcoholic wives of alcoholics. *Quarterly Journal of Studies on Alcohol, 20*, 77-85.

Jacobson, N. S. & Martin, M. B. (1976). Behavioral marriage therapy: Current status. *Psychological Bulletin, 83*, 540-557.

Jansen, C. (1977). Families in the treatment of alcoholism. *Journal of Studies on Alcohol, 38*, 114-130.

Johnson, V. E. (1973). *I'll quit tomorrow*. New York: Harper.

Keller, M. & Gerioli, C. (1976). Statistics on consumption of alcohol and alcoholism. Unpublished manuscript, *Journal of Studies on Alcohol*. New Brunswick, NJ.

Krimmel, H. (1971). *Alcoholism: Challenge for social work education*. New York: Council on Social Work Education.

Luks, A. (1983). *Will America sober up?* Boston, MA: Beacon Press.

Marlatt, G. A. (1982). Relapse prevention: A self-control program for the treatment of addictive behaviors. In R. B. Stuart (Ed.), *Adherence, compliance and generalization in behavioral medicine*. New York: Brunner/Mazel, 1982.

Maxwell, R. (1976). *The booze battle*. New York: Ballantine Books.

McCrady, B. S., Paolino, T. J., Longabaugh, R. & Rossi, J. (1979). Effects of joint hospital admission and couple's treatment for hospitalized alcoholics: A pilot study. *Addictive Behaviors, 4*, 155-167.

Meeks, D. E. & Kelly, C. (1970). Family therapy with families of recovering alcoholics. *Quarterly Journal of Studies on Alcohol, 31*, 399-413.

Olson, D. H. (1975). Marital and family therapy: A critical overview. In A. S. Gurman

& D. G. Rice (Eds.), *Couples in conflict: New directions in marital therapy*. New York: Jason Aronson.

Paolino, T. J. & McCrady, B. S. (1977). *The alcoholic marriage: Alternative perspectives*. New York: Grune & Stratton.

Prochaska, J. & Prochaska, J. (1978). Twentieth century trends in marriage and marital therapy. In T. J. Paolino & B. S. McCrady (Eds.), *Marriage and marital therapy: Psychoanalytic, behavioral and systems theory perspectives*. New York: Brunner/Mazel.

Scheiderer, E. G. & Bernstein, D. P. (1976). A case of chronic back pain and "unilateral" treatment of marital problems. *Journal of Behavior Therapy and Experimental Psychiatry, 7*, 47-50.

Selzer, M. L. (1971). The Michigan Alcoholism Screening Test (MAST): The quest for a new diagnostic instrument. *American Journal of Psychiatry, 3*, 176-181.

Stahmann, R. F. (1977). Treatment forms for marriage counseling. In R. F. Stahmann & W. J. Hiebert (Eds.), *Klemer's counseling in marital and sexual problems: A clinician's handbook*. 2nd ed.; Baltimore: Williams & Wilkins.

Steinglass, P. (1976). Experimenting with family treatment approaches to alcoholism, 1950-1975: A Review. *Family Process, 15*, 97-123.

Steinglass, P. (1978). The conceptualization of marriage from a systems theory perspective. In T. J. Paolino & B. S. McCrady (Eds.), *Marriage and marital therapy: Psychoanalytic, behavioral and systems theory perspectives*. New York: Brunner/Mazel.

Szapocznik, J., Kurtines, W. M., Foote, F. H., Perez-Vidal, A. & Hervis, O. (1983). Conjoint vs one person family therapy: Some evidence for the effectiveness of conducting family therapy through one person. *Journal of Consulting and Clinical Psychology, 51*, 889-899.

Thomas, E. J. (1984). *Designing interventions for the helping professions*. Beverly Hills, CA: Sage Publications.

Thomas, E. J. & Santa, C. A. (1982). Unilateral family therapy for alcohol abuse: A working conception. *The American Journal of Family Therapy, 10*, 49-60.

Thorne, D. R. (1983). Techniques for use in intervention. *Journal of Alcohol and Drug Education, 28*, 46-50.

Ward, R. F. & Faillace, L. A. (1970). The alcoholic and his helpers: A systems view. *Quarterly Journal of Studies on Alcohol, 31*, 684-691.

Zimberg, S. (1982). *The clinical management of alcoholism*. New York: Brunner/Mazel.

The Empirical Evaluation
of Clinical Practice:
A Survey of Four Groups
of Practitioners

James M. Cheatham

SUMMARY. Four groups of social work practitioners were studied to find out the extent to which they empirically evaluated their clinical practice, and to assess the conditions under which practitioners are likely to evaluate their practice. Data were collected by a self-administered mail questionnaire. Results showed that the group using a behavioral approach evaluated practice to a greater extent than members of the other three groups. It is claimed that single-subject methodology is most appropriate with behavioral interventions and that the steps in empirical practice evaluation are concomitantly the components of behavioral practice. Predictors of practice evaluation—client, agency, and practitioner factors—were found to be important in determining whether practitioners empirically evaluate their clinical practice. Closer coordination is recommended between schools of social work and agency field settings to determine both the competence and willingness of field supervisors and agency administrators to have empirical clinical practice conducted in their agencies.

INTRODUCTION

There has been increased discussion in the social work literature as to how best to evaluate clinical practice. One proposed solution to this question has been the integration of research procedures into the practice of social work through the use of single-

---

James M. Cheatham, PhD, PSC 4, Box 17264, APO San Francisco, CA 96408.
This article is based on the author's dissertation research.

subject methodology. The supporters of single-subject designs for the evaluation of clinical practice point to their practical feasibility for use in practice settings, the ability to provide clients and practitioners with continuous feedback on the therapeutic process, and their ability to identify cause-effect relationships by using clients as their own control (Bloom & Fischer, 1982; Hersen & Barlow, 1976; Jayaratne & Levy, 1979). Consequently, a primary focus in social work education during the past five years has been the integration of empirical practice into current models of direct practice (Barth, 1981; Berlin, 1983; Bloom & Fischer, 1982; Gambrill & Barth, 1980). Empirically based practice offers the practitioner a method of determining the impact of a particular intervention on a specified target problem in a precise, systematic and critical manner.

RESEARCH QUESTIONS

Despite the recent trend to train practitioners to engage in empirically based practice, little is known about the extent to which they actually use the methodology to evaluate their practice. Training in single-case evaluation methods does not automatically transfer to practice settings and appears to be related to other contingencies relative to the practitioner, the client, and the agency setting. Consequently, many educators and researchers have speculated about the reasons practitioners do not frequently use single-subject methods in their clinical practice, but there is lack of agreement about the specific reasons as to why single-subject designs are infrequently used.

The current thrust to produce scientist-practitioners in social work and the inherent difficulties related to this model of practice led to the design of a study to investigate two related research questions. The first question asks to what extent do different groups of social work practitioners empirically evaluate their clinical practice? While it is generally assumed that training in empirical practice methods will result in higher rates of evaluative activity among those trained in this technology, this assumption needs to be empirically tested. This study sampled two groups of social workers known to have been trained in idiographic research methods or presumed to use interventive techniques which incorporate components of empirical practice procedures. In addition, two groups of social work practitioners were sampled who were hypothesized to empirically evaluate practice to a lesser extent than the two groups trained in empirical practice methods.

The second research question asks, "What are the effects of client, agency and practitioner factors on the practice evaluation activities of social workers?" At this stage of development in the scientist-practitioner model, it is important to identify the conditions under which practitioners are likely to evaluate their practice. The willingness and ability of practitioners to use empirical research procedures in their clinical practice appears to be multi-determined. Identifying these variables is necessary to determine what changes in social work education, the agency context, or both are necessary in order to provide practitioners the necessary tools and environment to empirically evaluate their practice.

METHOD

Subjects

Four groups of social work practitioners were selected for study. As stated previously, two of the groups were known to have been trained in idiographic research methods or known to use interventive techniques which incorporate empirical practice procedures. One of these groups consisted of former graduate students from the School of Social Work, Florida State University who received training in idiographic research methods between 1980 and 1983. The second group consisted of the current members of the Social Work Group for the Study of Behavioral Methods. This group was self-identified by an interest in, or use of, behavioral techniques in direct practice activities. Two comparison groups were also used and consisted of a random sample of social workers listed in the 1982 *Register of Clinical Social Workers* and a sample of social work officers in the United States Air Force.

Procedure

Data were collected by a self-administered mail questionnaire that was sent to members of the four groups of social work practitioners described above. Of the 771 questionnaires mailed, 372 questionnaires were returned (48%). Of these 372 questionnaires, 317 were usable.

The eight page instrument used in this study was modeled after previous instruments used to evaluate the extent of practice evaluation activities, particularly those of Blythe (1983) and Gingerich (1984). The questionnaire sought information regarding the respondent's training in and knowledge of single-case methodology, as well as the respondent current use of the technology. In addition, questions were asked about the respondent's agency support regarding the empirical evaluation of clinical practice, characteristics of the respondent's practice and clients, as well as the practitioner's extent of agreement with integrating research procedures into clinical practice.

The dependent variable in this study was the amount of practice evaluation activity performed by the respondents and was measured by a series of 13 items associated with such activity. Higher scores indicate more frequent use of empirical practice procedures. Scores for each item could range from 0 = never performs the specific task to 5 = always performs the specific task. Practitioners were asked to indicate how often they performed such tasks as operationalizing the target problem and how often they used statistical techniques to evaluate client change. The scale is the EVALPRAC Scale developed by Blythe (1983). Coefficient alpha was used to assess the reliability of the scale and it was found that alpha = .86.

FINDINGS

Characteristics of the Practitioners

The average age of the 317 respondents was 38.71 years (*SD* = 9.7), with ages ranging from 23 to 68 years. About half (53%) of the sample was comprised of men, and 94.3% of the respondents ($n = 299$) were employed at the time they completed the questionnaire.

Over one-third of the respondents ($n = 117$) was employed in a mental health setting. Florida State University graduates were employed primarily in mental health and medical settings while members of the NASW group were employed primarily in mental health and private practice. Similarly, over two thirds (67.5%) of the U.S. Air Force group were employed in a mental health setting. In contrast, however, almost one-third (31.4%) of the Social Work Group for the Study of Behavioral Methods were employed in higher education settings with only 11% of this group indicating employment in a mental health setting.

For the entire sample, the social workers spent 53.3% of their time, on the average, engaged in direct practice activities. The percent of time spent in performing administrative or supervisory functions was 25.9%, while the percent of time involved in research activities was 5.1%. When comparing these statistics by group membership, as shown in Table 1, there were differences between the groups relative to time spent in the various activities. The members of the Social Work Group for the Study of Behavioral Methods spend, on the average, 30.9% of their time in direct practice activities as compared to almost twice this percent-

Table 1

Time Involved in Performance of Social Work Functions for

Total Sample by Group

Activity	Percent Total Sample (N=317)	Percent FSU (n=76)	Percent NASW (n=84)	Percent SWGSBM (n=35)	Percent USAF (n=77)
Direct Practice	57.3	63.8	58.5	30.9	60.6
Administration/ Supervision	25.9	24.1	28.6	27.8	22.8
Research	5.1	2.0	2.5	19.5	4.6
Other	11.5	10.1	10.4	21.7	11.5

Note. Group totals do not equal total sample size due to exclusion of respondents claiming membership in more than one group.

age of time by members of the Florida State, NASW and U.S. Air Force groups. In addition, members of the Social Work Group for the Study of Behavioral Methods spend, on the average, approximately one-fifth of their time engaged in research functions as compared to 2% for the Florida State University group, 2.5% for the NASW group, and 4.6% for the U.S. Air Force group. Time spent in research functions by the Social Work Group for the Study of Behavioral Methods was significantly different from the members of the three other groups ($F = 16.10$, df $= 3, 268$, p $< .001$, Eta square $= .15$).

One-third of the respondents (33.4%) described their approach as behavioral or cognitive-behavioral, and 62.9% of the Social Work Group for the Study of Behavioral Methods indicated that they used one of these two approaches. The percentage of social workers in the other three groups who used one of these two treatment approaches in their practice were as follows: 38.1% of the Florida State University group; 14.2% of the NASW group; and 33.8% of the U.S. Air Force group. Almost one-third (29.8%) of the NASW group identified their treatment approach as psychodynamic. The other most commonly identified treatment approach for all four groups was the "eclectic" category: 31.6% of the Florida State University group; 40.5% of the NASW group; 20% of the Social Work Group for the Study of Behavioral Methods; and 35.1% of the U.S. Air Force group.

Characteristics of Clients and Caseload

The average number of cases in a respondent's caseload was 33.9. For the four groups of interest in the study, the U.S. Air Force Group had the highest average caseload ($M = 42.9$) while the Social Work Group for the Study of Behavioral Methods had the lowest average caseload ($M = 25.0$). For all respondents, the largest percentage of cases (35.3%) were kept open between one and six months from the initial interview to termination. When comparing the four groups in the study, the Social Work Group for the Study of Behavioral Methods treats 65% of their clients in less than six months while the U.S. Air Force group treats 81.5% of their clients in less than six months. This finding is not surprising given the predominantly behavioral orientation of the Social Work Group for the Study of Behavioral Methods and the reported high caseload for the U.S. Air Force group.

Respondents were also asked to indicate what percentage of clients they felt were suitable for empirical practice procedures. For the total sample, the respondents indicated that on the average 41.4% (SD = 38.5) of their clients were suitable for empirical practice procedures. By group, the Social Work Group for the Study of Behavioral Methods indicated the highest percentage of suitable clients for empirical practice procedures (58.8%), while the NASW group indicated the lowest percentage, on the average, of client suitability for empirical practice procedures (36.1%). The percentage of clients suitable for empirical evaluation as indicated by the Florida State University and by the U.S. Air Force groups was 44.9% and 44.6%, respectively.

Respondents could also indicate what types of clients were deemed unsuitable for empirical practice procedures. As shown in Table 2, the type of client listed most frequently in terms of unsuitability for empirical practice was the client seen acutely for crisis intervention, followed by clients seen only for consultation/evaluation by the practitioner.

Agency Context for Practice Evaluation Activities

Respondents were asked to indicate how strongly they agreed (or disagreed) with a 16 item scale related to the agency context within which practice evaluation was conducted. Scores on these items could range from 5 = strongly agree to 1 = strongly disagree. Example items are "This agency provides sufficient time to conduct practice evaluation activities" and "This agency provides incentives for staff who evaluate their practice." The respondent's scores could be summed across the scale and used as a measure of the level of supportive contingencies that exist within the agency for practice evaluation activities. Coefficient alpha was used to assess the reliability of the scale and it was found that alpha = .93. There were significant differences between the mean scores on this scale for the four focal groups of the study. the Social Work Group for the Study of Behavioral

Table 2

Types of Clients Unsuitable for Empirical Practice Procedures

----

Type of Client	Number of Practioners Responding
Clients seen for acute support or crisis intervention only	27
Clients seen for consultation/evaluation	15
Clients seen for concrete or referral services	14
Psychotic Clients	13
Involuntary Clients	13
Clients with personality disorders	10
Chronically ill or terminally ill clients	9
Clients seen conjointly or in groups	7
Mentally retarded clients	5
Clients seeking insight	5
Suspicious clients	3
Noncompliant clients	2

Methods and the NASW group perceived their agency context, on the average, as being more supportive of the systematic evaluation of practice than the Florida State or U.S. Air Force groups ($F = 8.21$, df = 3,234, $p < .001$, Eta square = .0952).

The effects of environmental constraints, specifically the support or nonsupport of the agency toward empirical practice efforts, has been predicted to affect the extent to which empirical practice is conducted in the agency. Since single-subject designs are relatively new to the social work profession as a method of evaluating clinical practice, the effect of the environment on empirical practice needs ongoing examination.

Extent of Practice Evaluation Activity

Three indicators of practice evaluation activity were included in the questionnaire. The first was the total score from the EVALPRAC Scale (the criterion variable). The extent of practice evaluation activity among the four focal groups of the study was compared using analysis of variance procedures. Results of this analysis indicated that the Social Work Group for the Study of Behavioral Methods evaluated practice to a greater extent than members of the Florida State, NASW and U.S. Air Force groups (F = 7.33, df = 3,266, p < .001, Eta square = .0764). There were no significant differences among the Florida State, NASW and U.S. Air Force groups in terms of the extent of practice evaluation activity.

A second indicator of practice evaluation activity was a question asking respondents to indicate how often they had used both single-subject and group research designs within the past year. The number of social workers using each design and the average instance of use per worker are shown in Table 3. The single-subject design, pretest-posttest was used most often by workers (n = 52), followed by the AB design (n = 42). Across the four groups of interest in the study, the Social Work Group for the Study of Behavioral Methods had the highest percentage of social workers using each type of design with the exception of the single-subject design, pretest-posttest. The Florida State University group had the highest percentage of workers (31.0%) who used this design.

A third indicator of practice evaluation activity was an item asking respondents to indicate the approximate percentage of clients with whom they used single-subject or time series designs. On the average, all respondents reported using the technology with 14.7% of their clients. When comparing the four groups in the study, the Social Work Group for the Study of Behavioral Methods reported the highest percentage of empirical evaluation (35.6%) as compared with 10.4% for the FSU group; 14.5% for the NASW group; and 7.83% for the U.S. Air Force group.

Table 3

Use of Single-Subject and Group Research Designs for All

Respondents by Group

Type of Design	Number of Workers Using Designs and Mean Instance of Use Per Worker [a]				
	All Respondents	FSU	NASW	SWGSBM	USAF
Reversal Designs	22 (M=5.8)	4 (M=14.7)	1 (M=2.0)	10 (M=3.1)	1 (M=1.0)
AB Designs	42 (M=18.1)	11 (M=29.9)	6 (M=9.5)	15 (M=9.4)	4 (M=36)
B Designs	21 (M=5.4)	3 (M=9.0)	2 (M=11)	9 (M=2.8)	2 (M=1.0)
Multiple-Baseline Designs	34 (M=6.9)	9 (M=8.3)	5 (M=6.0)	12 (M=2.1)	3 (M=9.0)
Single-Subject Design Pretest-Posttest	52 (M=14.9)	13 (M=23.7)	10 (M=8.8)	10 (M=13.4)	9 (M=16.2)
Single-Group Design Pretest-Posttest	26 (M=7.9)	4 (M=3.0)	3 (M=6.0)	8 (M=5.1)	6 (M=3.3)
Experimental-Control Group Design, Pretest-Posttest	22 (M=6.0)	2 (M=1.0)	4 (M=2.3)	6 (M=1.2)	5 (M=9.8)
Other	9 (M=3.2)	1 (M=10.0)	1 (M=1.0)	6 (M=2.8)	1 (M=1.0)

Note. Group totals do not sum to the total sample size due to exclusion of respondents claiming membership in more than one group.

[a] Some workers used more than one type of design.

Practitioner, Client and Agency Effects on Empirical Practice Activity

Multiple regression analysis was used to address the relative effects of practitioner, client and agency variables on the extent of empirical practice evaluation activity. Each of 23 independent variables was tested for a significant association with the

EVALPRAC Scale with each variable being tested at the .006 level of significance in order to maintain the .05 experimentwise error rate. The following four variables had significant positive relationships with the EVALPRAC Scale: (1) practitioner agreement with integrating research procedures into clinical practice (F = 45.8, df = 1, 250, p < .001, R square change = .11367); (2) amount of coursework taken by the practitioner while in graduate school (F = 8.62, df = 1,250, p < .005, R square change = .02139); (3) the effectiveness of one's training in empirical clinical practice (F = 22.52, df = 1,250, p < .001, R square change = .05589); and (4) the level of supportive contingencies within the agency for the systematic evaluation of practice (F = 39.89, df = 1, 250, p < .001, R square change = .09900).

SUMMARY AND DISCUSSION

The finding that the Social Work Group for the Study of Behavioral Methods evaluated practice to a greater extent than members of the Florida State, NASW and U.S. Air Force groups was not surprising. It is claimed that single-subject methodology is most appropriate with behavioral interventions and that the steps in empirical practice evaluation are concomitantly the components of behavioral practice. Thus a behavioral approach was predicted to account for this group's significantly higher level of practice evaluation activity. An additional analysis was conducted to determine if group differences would disappear when treatment approach was held constant. This analysis of covariance showed that group differences on the EVALPRAC Scale remained after removing the effect of treatment orientation (F = 4.830, df = 3, 265, p < .003, Eta square = .05). Therefore, the behavioral orientation of the Social Work Group for the Study of Behavioral Methods did not account for the group differences.

In addition, on *a posteriori* analysis of the four groups was conducted relative to the significant predictor variables of practice evaluation activity that were identified in the regression analysis. This *a posteriori* analysis showed that the Social Work Group for the Study of Behavioral Methods had significantly more coursework and rated the effectiveness of their training in empirical clinical practice at significantly higher levels than either the NASW or U.S. Air Force groups. In addition, the Social Work Group for the Study of Behavioral Methods had significantly higher levels of agreement with integrating research procedures into clinical practice than the other three study groups ($F = 3.71$, df = 3, 262, p < .01, Eta square = .04). Finally, the Social Work Group for the Study of Behavioral Methods along with the NASW group perceived their agencies to be more supportive of practice evaluation activity than either the Florida State University or U.S. Air Force groups. These findings suggest that the predictors of practice evaluation activity identified by the multiple regression analysis may in fact play important roles in determining whether practitioners will empirically evaluate their clinical practice.

The four variables used to predict practice evaluation activity in the regression analysis warrant some further discussion. In regard to the practitioner's attitude toward the integration of research and practice, the design of the study (i.e., cross-sectional) does not permit one to know whether this attitude preceded training in empirical clinical practices or perhaps was a result of the training. The significance of this variable, however, highlights the need to maximize the possibility that research procedures are relevant to the social work practitioner. Rosenblatt (1968) found that clinicians did not regard research findings as being very relevant in solving the problems in day to day practice activities. Later studies (e.g., Rosen & Mutschler, 1982; Rosenblatt & Kirk, 1981) also concluded that social work research has not yet gained wide acceptance as to its relevance for clinical practice. The findings of this study suggest that alternative means must be considered for integrating research and practice in the social work curriculum and for teaching research methods to clinicians.

The importance of the agency environment in explaining empirical practice evaluation actively is only recently being investigated empirically (e.g., Blythe, 1983), but it has been referred to by numerous investigators in the field (Briar, 1980; Conte & Levy, 1980; Gingerich, 1984; Mutschler, 1984; Welch, 1983). It appears that failure to use empirical evaluation of clinical practice has usually focused on further educating the practitioner.

The need to train both field instructors and agency administrators as to the relevance of evaluating treatment outcomes empirically may be critically important. As discussed by Briar and Blythe (1985), consideration of how agency administrators can facilitate outcome evaluation needs to be given some priority vis-à-vis practice evaluation activity.

The findings that the amount of coursework in empirical clinical practice and the effectiveness of that training are significantly related to empirical practice evaluation come as no surprise. Although the relationship between evaluation activity and these two variables intuitively makes sense, one has to speculate about the ingredients of "effective training" since respondents were not asked to list the critical elements which they felt were related to the effectiveness of their training in empirical practice.

Based on the findings of this study, the following recommendations for both educational and research efforts can be made: (1) Given the significant relationship between the agency environment and the empirical evaluation of clinical practice, it would appear timely to conduct further experimental research within the agency setting vis à vis empirical clinical practice. Training practitioners to evaluate their practice in both supportive and nonsupportive environments would help determine with more specificity the salient agency variables that are most pertinent in terms of inhibiting or enhancing the ability to empirically evaluate practice. (2) Closer coordination is needed between schools of social work and agency field settings to determine both the competence and willingness of field supervisors and agency administrators to have empirical clinical practice conducted in their agencies. If agency personnel are indifferent or hostile to this method of practice evaluation, social work students who are interested in empirically evaluating their practice will experience both discouragement and a lack of priority for determining the outcome of any given intervention. (3) Ongoing experimental research is needed to compare various methods of training graduate students in order to determine the effectiveness of this training for both relevance and resultant knowledge. For example, Rabin (1985) suggests training clinical researchers in stages as a way of shaping their research skills in a manner similar to teaching clinical skills. (4) The issue of whether the empirical evaluation of clinical practice improves treatment outcome needs to be addressed through field research. The answer to this research question may perhaps be the best lever in persuading both practitioners and administrators to give priority to the empirical evaluation of practice. If it were found that empirical evaluation of practice enhances the quality of practice, the implications would be dramatic and apparent.

REFERENCES

Barth, R. P. (1981). Education for practice-research: Toward a reorientation. *Journal of Education for Social Work, 17,* 19-25.

Berlin, S. B. (1983). Single-case evaluation: Another version. *Social Work Research and Abstracts, 19,* 3-11.

Bloom, M. & Fischer, J. (1982). *Evaluating practice: Guidelines for the accountable professional.* Englewood Cliffs, NJ: Prentice Hall.

Blythe, B. J. (1983). An examination of practice evaluation among social workers. *Dissertation Abstracts International, 44,* 1952A-2607A. (University Microfilms No. 8326853).

Briar, S. (1980). Toward the integration of practice and research. In D. Fanshel (Ed.), *Future of social work research.* Washington, DC: National Association of Social Workers, Inc.

Briar, S. & Blythe, B. J. (1985). Agency support for evaluating the outcomes of social work services. *Administration in Social Work, 9,* 25-36.

Gambrill, E. D. & Barth, R. P. (1980). Single-case study designs revisited. *Social Work Research and Abstracts, 16,* 15-20.

Gingerich, W. J. (1984). Generalizing single-case evaluation from classroom to practice setting. *Journal of Education for Social Work, 20,* 74-82.

Hersen, M. & Barlow, D. H. (1976). *Single-case experimental designs.* New York: Pergamon Press.

Jayaratne, S. & Levy, R. L. (1979). *Empirical clinical practice.* New York: Columbia University Press.

Levy, R. L. (1981). On the nature of the clinical-research gap: The problems with some solutions. *Behavioral Assessment, 3,* 235-242.

Mutschler, E. (1984). Evaluating practice: A study of research utilization by practitioners. *Social Work, 29,* 332-337.

National Association of Social Workers, Inc. (1982). *NASW Register of Clinical Social Workers.* Silver Spring, MD: National Association of Social Workers.

Rabin, C. (1985). Matching the research seminar to meet practice needs: A method for integrating research and practice. *Journal of Social Work Education, 21,* 5-12.

Rosen, A. & Mutschler, E. (1982). Social work students' and practitioners' orientation to research. *Journal of Education for Social Work, 18,* 62-68.

Rosenblatt, A. (1968). The practitioner's use and evaluation of research. *Social Work, 13,* 53-59.

Rosenblatt, A. & Kirk, S. A. (1981). Cumulative effect of research courses on knowledge and attitudes of social work students. *Journal of Education for Social Work,* *17,* 26-34.

Welch, G. J. (1983). Will graduates use single-subject designs to evaluate their case-work practice? *Journal of Education for Social Work, 19,* 42-46.

Medical Social Work Management of Urinary Incontinence in the Elderly: A Behavioral Approach

Elsie M. Pinkston
Michael W. Howe
Donald K. Blackman

SUMMARY. The effect of stimulus cues and social reinforcement on urinary incontinence of three wheel-chair bound, nursing home residents was investigated using a multiple-baseline across subjects. The residents included three seriously impaired elderly women who were offered the opportunity to use the toilet hourly and taken to the toilet on a 2-hour schedule. Praise and cookies were provided as a consequence for appropriate urination in the toilet. Following the intervention opportunities for toileting increased, and there was a decrease in urinary incontinence, and an increase in appropriate urinary toileting.

Urinary incontinence is a serious bio-social concern of many elderly people and their families. In the community, the incontinent elderly may be excluded from social interaction with their families and friends, and incontinence is one of the highest causes of long term institutional placement (Portnoi, 1981; Ouslander, 1983). In long-term care institutions, the incontinent elderly may also be considered socially unacceptable and systematically excluded from social and potentially therapeutic activities,

---

The authors are with the School of Social Service Administration, The University of Chicago.

and are more likely to suffer serious irritations (Ouslander, Kane & Abrass, 1982).

Behavioral research which employs both respondent and operant frameworks has proved successful for increasing continence. The "bell-and-pad method" developed by Mowrer and Mowrer (1938) and modified by Crosby (1950) and Lovibond (1964) has been used to treat childhood enuresis (Yates, 1970; Atthowe, 1973). Several operant studies have reduced incontinence of mentally deficient inpatients (Dayon, 1964; Giles & Wolf, 1966; Azrin & Foxx, 1971; Foxx & Azrin, 1973), as well as of children in home environments (Mahoney, Van Wagenen & Meyerson, 1971; Azrin & Foxx, 1974).

In spite of the widespread success of the behavioral treatment of incontinence with some populations, only a few studies have reported the extension of these methods to older people. Of these studies, four have involved institutionalized adult subjects without organic involvement, and have reported successful outcomes (Carpenter & Simon, 1960; Monroe, 1963; Wetzel, 1969; Wagner & Paul, 1970). Few studies however, involving organic brain impairment of the elderly have demonstrated improved urinary incontinence (Atthowe, 1972; Schnelle et al., 1983), and some studies involving day-time incontinence with an organically impaired, institutionalized population (Grosicki, 1968; Pollock & Liberman, 1974) have shown no improvement.

Pollack & Liberman (1974) used candy and cigarettes as consequences for continence but made no provision in their treatment program to systematically reinforce proper toileting responses. They found that delivering candy and cigarettes on a fixed-interval schedule for being dry would not increase continence; they stated that the missing link in their program was to assume "that the subject would connect bathroom usage with dry pants and in order to decrease wet pants he would increase bathroom usage" (Pollack & Liberman, 1974, p. 490).

Other treatment procedures have included the following: 2-hour toileting with verbal approval for eliminating successfully (Carpenter & Simon, 1960); changing clients into green fatigues after incontinence as a punishment contingency (Carpenter & Simon, 1960); encouraging proper urination before sleep, and waking subjects every three hours for toileting (Monroe, 1963);

interacting socially with subjects, contingent upon dryness (Grosicki, 1968; Pollack & Liberman, 1974); using tokens in exchange for dryness and eliminating properly (Grosicki, 1969; Atthowe, 1972); using a combination of the "bell-and-pad" method with contingent presentation of candy, cigarettes, meals, and praise (Wagner & Paul, 1970); and hourly checks and prompts, with social approval for dry checks and disapproval for wet checks (Schnelle et al., 1983).

This research represents an application of the social worker/researcher model of intervention in which intervention, social work values, and research methodology are combined to solve an important client problem. While urinary incontinence has not usually been defined as a social work problem, it is of major importance in humane care and well within the fundamental commitment to the total bio-social welfare of individuals that is the purview of medical social work.

The purpose of this study was to analyze and behaviorally treat the problem of urinary incontinence with subjects who were wheelchair-bound and diagnosed as organically brain damaged. The primary interest was to analyze the effect of the treatment package, which included reinforcing both dryness and toileting behavior. In addition, the authors analyzed the effectiveness with which treatment variables were implemented.

Three factors distinguished this study from the previous studies of incontinence with the elderly: (1) the unique characteristics of the sample population, (2) the system of treatment intervention, and (3) the strategy of the research design.

METHOD

Setting and Subjects

This study was conducted by social worker/researchers in a long-term care facility for the aged with approximately 230 residents. The subjects were drawn from the thirty female residents occupying the fifth floor. Generally, the self-care capacities of these residents were minimal, and they required more staff attention than residents of other units of the home. The nurses' aides

and the orderly were primarily responsible for helping these residents without self-care functions.

The authors used the following criteria to select three subjects:

1. The subject must be incontinent.
2. The incontinence must not be due to an acute or transient
   medical process.
3. The subject must be over 65 years of age.
4. The subject must be wheelchair-bound.
5. The subject must have been a resident of the home for at
   least one year prior to the beginning of the study.

Physical impairments were noted and monitored medically,
but subjects were not eliminated from the sample because of
chronic brain or genito-urinary system impairments. Three residents on the fifth floor fulfilled these requirements and served as
the study sample. All were female and have lived in the home
from 1 to 3 years, and agreed to participate in the study. Because
of their impaired state, permission was also obtained from the
Director who served as their guardian.

Subject *one* (S1) was 77 years old, and medically diagnosed as
having possible organic brain syndrome, hypertension, osteoporosis, and osteoarthritis. Because she was unable to use a
walker, S1 had been confined to a wheelchair by the medical
staff 3 months prior to the study. At the time of the study, she
could transfer from wheelchair to toilet only with assistance, and
still after 3 months of physical therapy, she could not adequately
propel a wheelchair. When admitted to the home, S1 complained
of urinating frequently (with no history of hematuria or dysuria),
but was evidently continent when admitted. Because residents
complained of her incontinence in the main dining hall, S1 was
restricted to the fifth floor dining room. When questioned by
staff about her inability to stay dry, S1 would adamantly deny
being incontinent.

Subject *two* (S2) was 79 years old, and medically diagnosed as
having organic brain syndrome, generalized arteriosclerosis with
a history of strokes, osteoporosis of spine, collapse of lumbar
vertebrae, and incontinence. S2 could operate a wheelchair but
could not transfer to and from it independently. At the time of the

study, she had had urinary incontinence for over 2 years; she reported no awareness of micturition, and previous bowel and bladder programs had proved unsuccessful.

Subject *three* (S3) was 94 years old, with the medical diagnoses of organic brain syndrome, arteriosclerotic heart disease with episodes of left ventricle failure, generalized arteriosclerosis, and partial deafness. S3 could not propel a wheelchair or self-transfer. She was incontinent when admitted and at the time of the study was incapable of talking coherently, although she maintained receptive language.

Observation and Reliability Procedures

Urinary incontinence was defined as any bladder elimination occurring while on the unit in which a subject did not use appropriate toileting facilities. The obvious sign of eliminating was wet or soiled clothing, and/or bedding, or urine on the floor near the wheelchair.

The observer, seated in a chair halfway between two bathrooms, was equipped with a stopwatch, a notebook, and data sheets, recorded wetness or dryness, clothes changing, and toileting of subjects. From 7:00 a.m. to 3:00 p.m., 5 days per week, all subjects were unobtrusively observed. The observer recorded whenever subjects entered and used toileting facilities or had their clothes changed. Every 15 minutes subjects were recorded as being either wet or dry. These observations provided data on daytime incontinence, on initiation, frequency, and duration of toileting, and on the clothes changing of subjects.

While the major focus of the study was on daytime incontinence, nocturnal incontinence was monitored as well. Each night the 11:00 p.m.-7:00 a.m. nursing staff recorded bedding changes in their nursing notes. The nursing notes provided a gross permanent record of subjects' nighttime wetness or dryness.

Observations were recorded on the nursing staff's accuracy in carrying out wetness/dryness and toileting sequences. The nursing staff's conduct was observed by the independent observer during the wetness/dryness and toileting sequences of the treatment program, and each sequence was rated for staff response to the timer-alarm, and appropriate staff response to the alarm. (Behavioral codes can be obtained from E. Pinkston.) Each observation day, four toileting and four wetness/dryness sequences were observed and rated.

Subject interactions with staff and other residents were also monitored. Because there were no changes in total social interactions, staff social interactions, or resident social interactions with subjects between baseline and treatment, the observation methods are not presented.

Reliability

Interobserver reliability estimates were recorded on independent and dependent variables. The independent observers' records were then compared for agreement and disagreement and interobserver reliability was calculated. Reliability on nocturnal incontinence was obtained by an independent observer who made bedding checks before beds were changed in the morning. Reliability was calculated by comparing records with the nursing notes for agreement and disagreement. The percentage agreement between observers was calculated from these observational records as follows:

$$\text{Interobserver Reliability} = \frac{\text{Number of Observer Agreements}}{\text{Number of Observer Agreements} + \text{Number of Observer Disagreements}}$$

Experimental Design

This research employed a multiple-baseline design using three subjects to evaluate the treatment program (Baer, Wolf & Risley, 1968; Hersen & Barlow, 1976; Howe, 1974; Sidman, 1960). This design was especially appropriate for treating urinary incontinence since reversing treatment was considered undesirable.

TREATMENT: PROCEDURES

The treatment procedures consisted of two alternating schedules of reinforcement: (1) a wetness/dryness sequence on a fixed-interval, 2-hour schedule and (2) a toileting sequence on a fixed-interval, 2-hour schedule. The nurses' aides primarily responsible for the treatment program made observations and recorded their activities in the wetness/dryness and toileting sequences during treatment conditions.

Wetness/Dryness Sequence

Every day at 8:30 a.m., 10:30 a.m., 12:30 p.m., 2:30 p.m., 4:30 p.m., 6:30 p.m., and 8:30 p.m., a Westclox (Model 50045) alarm clock placed at the central nurses' station signaled nurses' aides to make a wetness/dryness check. Nurses' aides were instructed to check the subject's clothing and, if wet, to say nothing to the subject and simply record the fact on the wetness/dryness checksheet provided. If the subject was dry, the nurses' aide was instructed to record the fact and to praise the subject lavishly for being dry.

Toileting Sequence

At the beginning of the treatment conditions, each subject's wheelchair was equipped with a Westinghouse ("Baby Ben" Model 11037) alarm clock which was set to ring at 2-hour intervals. The purpose of the apparatus was discussed with subjects individually; they were told that when the alarm sounded, a nurses' aide would come and take them to the toilet. The sound of the timer-alarm set the occasion for toileting for both subjects and staff.

This alarm was set and reset at 2-hour intervals — 7:30 a.m., 9:30 a.m., 11:30 a.m., and 1:30 p.m. — at which times the subject was taken to the toilet regardless of wetness or dryness at that particular moment. However, if the subject was dry, the nurses' aide was instructed to praise the subject before bringing the subject to the toileting facility. Before the subject was transferred to the toilet, a 4-inch-square piece of blue litmus paper, a reliable measure of the presence of urine, was placed in the toilet bowl.

Then, depending on the subject's physical capabilities, the subject was helped on the toilet. If the litmus paper turned pink, the nurses' aide praised the subject while helping her back into the wheelchair and offered the subject a snack. If the subject did not void, the nurses' aide simply helped the subject back into the wheelchair with minimal interaction. Finally, if at any time the subject requested toileting, the nurses' aided promptly complied; even so, when the alarm rang, the subject was taken to the toilet again.

The toileting checksheet was filled out after each toileting sequence. On the checksheet, the nurses' aides recorded the time, whether or not the subject voided, whether or not they praised the subject and offered her a snack, whether or not the subject accepted the snack, and any comments they wished to make.

STAFF TRAINING AND SUPERVISION

While the nursing staff was informed that a study would be undertaken on resident incontinence, they were not told (by prior mutual agreement) exactly how the program would be conducted, which residents would participate, or what their own specific roles in the program would be until after stable baseline rates were obtained. At that time, a special staff meeting was called in which the staff procedures were read and the wetness/dryness and toileting sequences and records were discussed. The staff was told that a copy of the staff procedures, along with recording forms for the wetness/dryness and toileting sequences, would be kept at the nurses' station and that a supply of litmus paper would be kept in the toileting facilities.

No formal or informal training in learning theory or behavior modification was introduced in this or in subsequent meetings. The procedures and the residents' and staffs' reactions to the procedures were discussed during weekly floor staff meetings. With the exception of understaffed days, a nurses' aide was assigned to conduct the procedures with individual subjects. Staff members were infrequently prompted when alarms could not be heard because staff were on the floor doing errands. Finally, on approximately 30% of treatment days, the social worker toileted

S3, because of S3's excessive weight and a lack of staff appropriate for the task.

RESULTS

Figure 1 contains the frequency of daytime incontinence before and during treatment for S1, S2 and S3. In each case, after introducing treatment was introduced, there was a systematic decrease in the incidence of urinary incontinence. After day 21 for S1, day 39 for S2 and 51 for S3, the frequency of incontinence markedly decreased.

During a 29-day baseline period, S1 soiled her clothing on 26 days. S1's incontinence ranged from 0 to 5 incidents per day, and on just less than half of these baseline days, she soiled her clothing more than twice per day (within a single 8-hour observation period). The treatment program was introduced for a total of 46 observation days (approximately nine weeks). S1 was completely dry on 36 of these treatment days and did not soil her clothing more than twice in one observation day. Therefore, a substantial decrease in incontinence had occurred. The decrease was immediately apparent and was maintained throughout the treatment phase of the study.

During the 38-day baseline period, S2 soiled her clothing on 34 days. On 25 of these 38 baseline days, she was incontinent two or more times a day. The day-to-day frequency of S2's incontinence varied considerably, ranging from 0 to 7 (within a daily 8-hour observation period) before the treatment program was begun. The treatment program was introduced for a total of 36 observation days. While on 24 of the 36 treatment days, or three-fourths of the treatment days, S2 was completely dry, this client was slower to respond to the program than the other subjects. She soiled her clothing 12 of the 36 treatment days, nine of which occurred during the first 18 days, only three during the last 18 days. A decrease in incontinence had occurred, but not as immediately; once the daily frequency of incontinence was reduced, the decrease was maintained for the duration of the study.

Of the three subjects in the study, S3 had the lowest but most consistent initial frequency of incontinence. During a 50-day baseline period (approximately two and one-half months), S3

188   *PROGRESS IN BEHAVIORIAL SOCIAL WORK*

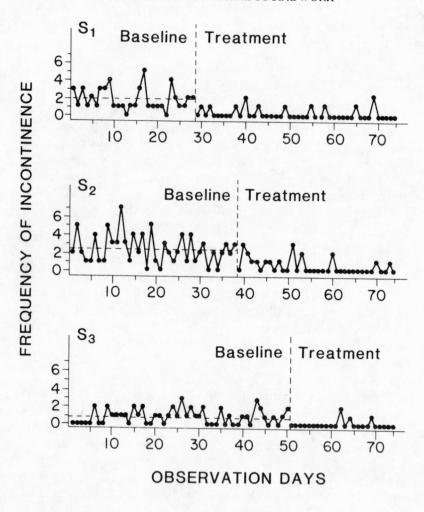

FIGURE 1. Daily frequency of incontinence across days observed.

soiled her clothing on 30 days. S3's incontinence ranged from 0 to 3 incidents per day, but on only 12 of 50 days did she soil her clothing twice or more in one day. The treatment program was introduced for a total of 24 observation days (approximately 5 weeks). S3 was completely dry on 21 of these treatment days. On only one occasion during this time did she soil her clothing more than once in one day. An immediate and systematic decrease occurred and the treatment gain was maintained throughout the study.

Figure 2 contains the percentage of complete days dry, as well as the average incidence of incontinence during baseline and treatment for S1, S2, and S3. It was demonstrated that there were consistent increases in the percentage of days completely dry with all subjects. S1 was dry on 7% of the days during baseline, increasing to 78% during treatment; S2 was dry on 11% of the days during baseline, increasing to 67% during treatment; S3 was dry on 40% of the days during baseline and reached 88% during treatment. These represent improvements of 71, 56, and 48 percentage points between baseline and treatment for S1, S2 and S3.

The average daily incidence of incontinence, also shown in Figure 2, demonstrated consistent and marked decreases between baseline and treatment with all three subjects. During baseline, S1 and S2 soiled their clothing approximately twice per day (average of 1.88 and 2.4, respectively), while S3 soiled her clothing once per day (average of .88). After the treatment program was introduced, S1 soiled herself only 10 times during 46 treatment days or approximately once every 4 to 5 days; S2 soiled herself 12 times during 36 treatment days or approximately once every 3 days; while S3 soiled herself 3 times during 21 days, or approximately once every 7 days. These results clearly demonstrate that a systematic and marked decrease in the incidence of incontinence was obtained when the treatment program was introduced.

The frequency of toileting can be seen in Figure 3 during baseline and treatment for each subject. All subjects were toileted an average of once per day during baseline. These data were also analyzed to compare the percentage of days during baseline and treatment in which subjects were toileted; S1 was toileted on 61% of the days during baseline and 100% during treatment; S2 was toileted 76% of the days during baseline and 100% during treatment; and finally, S3 was toileted on 54% of the days during baseline and 100% of the days during treatment.

A comparison of Figure 3 with Figure 1 baselines shows that, on one day for S1 and on 8 days for S3, subjects were not toi-

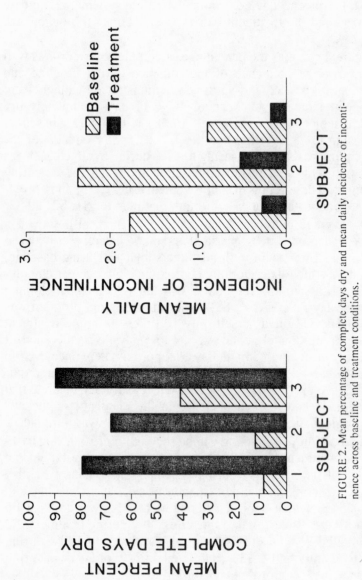

FIGURE 2. Mean percentage of complete days dry and mean daily incidence of incontinence across baseline and treatment conditions.

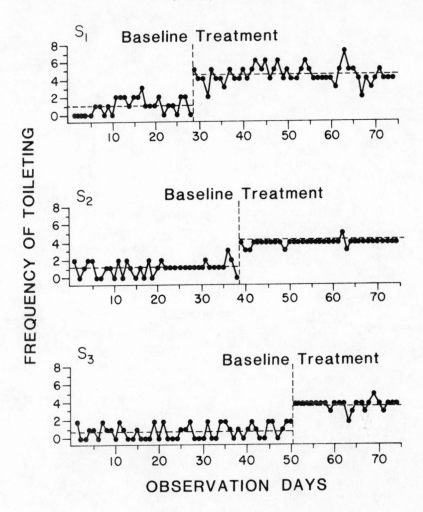

FIGURE 3. Daily frequency of toileting across days observed.

leted, yet they were not observed to be incontinent. Incontinence may not have been observed because subjects did not urinate (e.g., on a day of extremely low fluid intake), subjects dribbled urine into an incontinence pad which could not be observed, subjects urinated while off the floor, or (while extremely unlikely) subjects urinated but were not seen by the observer.

DISCUSSION

Clearly, these treatment procedures increased staff efforts to toilet wheelchair bound individuals and decreased the incontinent behaviors of the resident subjects. Further, subjects were required to spend less time in the bathroom sitting on the toilet although they were offered the opportunity to be taken more often and did increase their appropriate toilet behavior.

During the study it was apparent that one of the reasons staff did not use at least a 2-hour toilet procedure was that they did not believe it would work. In this respect, the data demonstrated to the staff and administration alike that incontinence of many wheelchair-bound elderly with organic brain disorders need not be an irreversible fact of life. The environmental influence of a clear cue in stimulating staff behavior, even under circumstances where they were skeptical of the effectiveness of the procedure, was positive.

These urinary incontinence management procedures, when used with seriously mentally and physically impaired individuals, represent a part of a prosthetic environment for maintaining the highest level of functioning possible. Therefore, the procedures are not a cure for urinary incontinence but instead, are a way of maximizing continent behavior that must be continued in order to effectively maintain high rates of staff toileting behavior and low rates of resident urinary incontinence.

A limitation of this study is that it is not possible to generalize the results to all wheelchair-bound elderly individuals. It should be noted, however, that these clients were identified by the staff as the worst cases of incontinence of the non-bedridden clients.

A further improvement of this procedure would be to determine the appropriate toileting interval for each individual from their baseline of incontinence. It is possible that hourly prompts are not necessary for all residents. In ambulatory individuals, bladder capacities differ as well as the presence of the internal physical cues for the need to urinate. These issues suggest the use of individual analysis when possible. It is also reasonable to assume that the reinforcement of appropriate toilet behavior is more relevant than reinforcement of dry pants, i.e., reinforcing the desired response rather than the result.

Although these procedures are not for all incontinence problems, they have important implications for establishing routines in nursing home care. Further, the modification of staff behavior seems more humane and in keeping with good hygiene than staff behavior patterns in which there is no routine toilet schedule.

REFERENCES

Atthowe, J. M. (1972). Controlling nocturnal enuresis in severely disabled chronic patients. *Behavior Therapy, 3*, 232-239.

Atthowe, J. M. (1973). Nocturnal enuresis and behavior therapy: A functional analysis. In R. D. Rubin, J. P. Brady & J. D. Henderson (Eds.), *Advances in behavior therapy*. New York: Academic Press.

Azrin, N. H. & Fox, R. M. (1971). A rapid method of toilet training the institutionalized retarded. *Journal of Applied Behavior Analysis, 4*, 89-99.

Azrin, N. H. & Fox, R. M. (1974). *Toilet training in less than a day*. New York: Simon and Schuster.

Baer, D. M., Wolf, M. M. & Risley, T. R. (1969). Some current dimensions of applied behavior analysis. *Journal of Applied Behavior Analysis, 1*, 91-97.

Carpenter, H. A. & Simon, R. (1960). The effect of several methods of training on long-term incontinence, behaviorally regressed hospitalized psychiatric patients. *Nursing Research, 9*, 17-22.

Crosby, N. D. (1950). Essential enuresis: Successful treatment based on physiological concepts. *Medical Journal of Australia, 2*, 533-543.

Dayon, M. (1964). Toilet training retarded children in a state residential institution. *Mental Retardation, 2*, 116-117.

Fox, R. M. & Azrin, N. H. (1973). *Toilet training the retarded*. Champaign, IL.: Research Press.

Giles, D. K. & Wolf, M. M. (1966). Toilet training institutionalized, severe retardates: An application of behavior modification techniques. *American Journal of Mental Deficiency, 70*, 766-780.

Grosicki, J. P. (1968). Effect of operant conditioning on modification of incontinence in neuro-psychiatric geriatric patients. *Nursing Research, 17*, 304-311.

Hersen, M. & Barlow, D. (1976). *Single case experimental designs: Strategies for studying behavior change*. New York: Pergamon Press.

Howe, M. W. (1974). Casework self-evaluation: A single-subject approach. *Social Service Review, 48*, 1-23.

Lovibond, S. H. (1964). *Conditioning and enuresis*. Oxford: Pergamon.

Mahoney, K., Van Wagenen, R. K. & Meyerson, B. (1971). Toilet training of normal and retarded children. *Journal of Applied Behavior Analysis, 4*, 173-181.

Monroe, K. L. (1963). Treatment of nocturnal enuresis among hospitalized neuropsychiatric patients. Unpublished doctoral dissertation, Purdue University, Hammond, Indiana.

Mowrer, O. H. & Mowrer, W. A. (1938). Enuresis: A method for its study and treatment. *American Journal of Orthopsychiatry, 8*, 436-447.

Ouslander, J. G. (1983). Incontinence and nursing homes: Epidemiology and management. *The Gerontologist, 23* speical issue), 257.

Ouslander, J. G., Kane, R. L. & Abrass, J. B. (1982). Urinary incontinence in elderly home patients. *Journal of the American Medical Association, 248*, 1194-1198.

Pollack, D. D. & Liberman, R. P. (1974). Behavior therapy of incontinence in demented inpatients. *The Gerontologist, 14*, 488-491.

Portnoi, V. A. (1981). Urinary incontinence in the elderly. *American Family Physician, 23*, 151-154.

Schnelle, J. F., Traughber, B., Morgan, D. B., Embry, J. E., Binion, F. & Coleman, A. (1983). Management of geriatric incontinence in nursing home. *Journal of Applied Behavior Analysis, 16*, 235-241.

Sidman, M. (1960). *Tactics of scientific research*. New York: Basic Books.

Wagner, B. R. & Paul, G. L. (1970). Reduction of incontinence in chronic mental patients: A pilot project. *Journal of Behavior Therapy and Experimental Psychiatry, 1*, 29-38.

Wetzel, L. C. (1969). The effects of operant conditioning and nico-metrzol on the modification of daytime incontinence of regressed chronic schizophrenics. Unpublished doctoral dissertation, University of Illinois, Chicago, Illinois.